NAVIGATE THE COMPLEXITIES OF EARLY-ONSET DEMENTIA

UNDERSTANDING SYMPTOMS AND FINDING SOLUTIONS

JEFF HOLLITZ

TABLE OF CONTENTS

Introduction   7

1. UNDERSTANDING EARLY-ONSET DEMENTIA   11
   Defining Early-Onset Dementia: Symptoms and Diagnosis   12
   The Emotional Journey: Accepting a Diagnosis of Early-Onset   14
   Biological Insights: How Early-Onset Dementia Affects the Brain   16
   Differentiating Early-Onset from Later-Onset Dementia   18
   Early Signs and When to Seek a Professional Opinion   21

2. LEGAL AND FINANCIAL PLANNING   27
   Drafting a Living Will: A Step-by-Step Guide   28
   Understanding and Setting up Durable Power of Attorney   31
   Financial Planning Strategies for Early-Onset Dementia   33
   Navigating Insurance and Benefits for Younger Patients   35
   Protecting Assets and Planning for Long-Term Care Needs   37

3. DAILY LIFE ADJUSTMENTS   39
   Modifying Your Home for Safety and Accessibility   39
   Effective Communication Strategies as Dementia Progresses   42
   Managing Work-Life after Diagnosis   44
   Nutrition and Physical Health: Best Practices   47
   Technology and Tools to Support Independence   51

4. EMOTIONAL AND PSYCHOLOGICAL
    SUPPORT   55
    Dealing with Grief and Emotional Turmoil
    Post-Diagnosis   56
    Support Systems: Building and Maintaining
    Relationships   59
    Techniques for Managing Caregiver Stress and
    Avoiding Burnout   61
    Counseling and Therapy Options for Families   64
    The Role of Support Groups in Emotional
    Well-Being   67

5. PRACTICAL CAREGIVING STRATEGIES   71
    Establishing Effective Routines for Patients and
    Caregivers   71
    Navigating Behavioral Changes and Challenges   74
    Activities of Daily Living: Tips for Facilitating
    Independence   78
    The Importance of Personalized Patient-
    Centered Care   79
    Respite Care: Understanding Its Importance
    and How to Access It   81

6. ENHANCING QUALITY OF LIFE   85
    Therapeutic Activities Suitable for Early-Onset
    Dementia   85
    Social Engagement: Keeping Connected with
    the Community   90
    Physical Exercise and Its Benefits to Cognitive
    Health   93
    Planning for Meaningful Outings and Visits   97

7. ADVANCED CARE PLANNING   101
    Understanding and Preparing for the Later
    Stages of Dementia   101
    When to Consider Memory Care Facilities   104
    Palliative Care Options and Discussions   107
    End-of-Life Care: Making Decisions with
    Dignity   109
    The Role of Hospice in Managing Advanced
    Dementia   111

8. ADVOCACY AND COMMUNITY
   INVOLVEMENT   115
   Becoming a Dementia Advocate: Steps and
   Strategies   116
   Using Social Media to Connect and Educate
   Others   119
   Organizing Community Events and
   Fundraisers   121
   The Importance of Participating in Research   125
   Legislative Advocacy: How You Can Influence
   Dementia Care Policies   127

9. RESOURCES AND CONTINUING SUPPORT   131
   Comprehensive Directory of Resources for
   Early-Onset Dementia   131
   Continuing Education: Opportunities for
   Learning and Growth   134
   Innovations in Dementia Care: Keeping Up-to-
   Date   136
   Building a Sustainable Caregiving Network   140
   The Future of Dementia Care: Trends and
   Predictions   143
   Reviewing and Revising Care Plans: An
   Ongoing Process   145
   Nurturing Hope and Positivity in the Face of
   Dementia   147
   Reflections and Next Steps for Caregivers and
   Patients   150

   Conclusion   153
   Bibliography   157

INTRODUCTION

It's not always like the movies make it out to be. One day, you're on the way to dinner and notice that they forgot their keys or stumbled over remembering your name, and you think nothing of it. A few months later, you look back in hindsight as the changes have progressed and realize that something is going on—something like dementia. It's a heartbreaking and life-altering realization to know that a loved one is no longer able to follow along or care for themselves, sometimes the very same loved one who raised or cared for you.

This is how my journey with dementia began—a slow roll toward the inevitable point where we couldn't ignore it anymore, and then the effects of reaching that point. When my grandfather was diagnosed with dementia, two things happened: The last several months suddenly made perfect sense, and my family irreparably changed.

This might be exactly how you're feeling right now. You might be confused, scared, or worried for your loved one, and the question of "What's next?" has never been stronger in your mind. Or, maybe it's yourself that you're worried about, as noticing the onset of dementia in your own life is never something easy to digest. It's completely normal to feel this way, and if you're not sure what to do or where to go from here, don't worry—you're not alone.

This book focuses on early-onset dementia, a term that you might have heard but aren't really sure what it means. Distinct from the types of dementia that typically affect people later in life, early-onset dementia can begin as early as your thirties, forties, or fifties. This book is here to guide you through an in-depth understanding of dementia, whether you're here for yourself, a loved one, or someone else that you care for. It's your copilot in navigating the complex journey that lies ahead.

Here, we are going to cover a range of topics together, from the medical explanations of early-onset dementia to the everyday practicalities of caregiving. You will find stories from other families, advice from medical professionals, and the latest research findings. Together, these elements create a unique blend of personal experience and expert knowledge that will guide you in navigating such a tumultuous time. Empathy, encouragement, and depth are what you can expect to find here.

The understanding of early-onset dementia that you will find here is crucial, not just for providing care but for fostering an environment where empathy flourishes. The insights and strategies shared here mean you can make a significant difference in the lives of those affected, be it yourself or someone you love.

Thank you for your courage to learn more and your dedication to supporting your loved ones or yourself. Let this book serve as your guide and companion, inspiring you to take action and remain hopeful in the face of challenges. Together, we can improve the lives of those dealing with early-onset dementia, ensuring they feel valued and loved every step of the way.

1

UNDERSTANDING EARLY-ONSET DEMENTIA

Have you ever found yourself in a room wondering why you were even there or started a task only to forget what you were doing halfway through? For many, these moments are just blips, easily laughed off. But when incidents like these become frequent and disrupt daily life, they can signal something more profound—perhaps early-onset dementia. While forgetfulness can be a part of normal aging, the patterns seen in early-onset dementia are different, often more pervasive and impactful even in younger adults.

This chapter delves into the specifics of early-onset dementia to provide you with a clear understanding of what it is, the symptoms it presents, and the diagnostic processes involved. This initial understanding is vital when it comes to identifying and managing this condition effectively, thus improving quality of life and providing a foundation for better-informed decisions.

DEFINING EARLY-ONSET DEMENTIA: SYMPTOMS AND DIAGNOSIS

Early-onset dementia refers to dementia that occurs before the age of 65 ("What Are the Signs of Alzheimer's Disease?" n.d.). It's a broad term that covers many forms of dementia, including Alzheimer's disease, vascular dementia, frontotemporal dementia, and more. Understanding early-onset dementia is essential because it highlights a critical point: Dementia does not only affect the elderly. In recognizing this, we can better address the unique challenges and needs that younger people with dementia face.

The symptoms of early-onset dementia can vary significantly but often include memory loss that disrupts daily activities, challenges in planning or solving problems, difficulty completing familiar tasks at home or work, confusion with time or place, and changes in mood or personality. For example, someone who was once very punctual and detail-oriented might start missing deadlines and forgetting important dates. Unlike typical age-related changes, such as occasionally forgetting names or appointments, early-onset dementia involves more frequent, consistent, and severe lapses (Mayo Clinic 2023).

Diagnosing early-onset dementia involves a comprehensive evaluation, usually by a general practitioner and then by a professional trained to manage dementia and related concerns. An evaluation for early-onset dementia typically includes medical history, physical examinations, neurological tests, and mental status assessments. Brain imaging tests like MRI and CT scans are also used to rule out other causes of symptoms, such as tumors or stroke, and to detect changes that are indicative of dementia (NHS 2023). The process can be lengthy and complex, and it's because symptoms like these are often attributed to stress or depression, especially in younger people ("Is It Dementia or Depression?" 2021). Being so thorough means that medical professionals can help ascertain a more accurate diagnosis.

It's good to receive a diagnosis at all, but it's great to receive a diagnosis as early on as possible. Recognizing early-onset dementia early on can open the door to management strategies that may help slow the progression of symptoms and improve quality of life. This also allows for better planning for the future, including financial planning, career adjustments, and family dynamics. Early diagnosis provides people with dementia and their families more opportunities to make informed choices about care, treatments, and personal or legal matters that could become more challenging as the disease progresses.

Reflective Journaling

Take a moment to reflect on the symptoms we've discussed so far. If you or someone you know is experiencing similar patterns, consider noting them down in a journal along with the setting and date of that instance. A record like this can be helpful when consulting with healthcare providers, as it provides a clear picture of what has been occurring over time.

THE EMOTIONAL JOURNEY: ACCEPTING A DIAGNOSIS OF EARLY-ONSET

The moment a diagnosis of early-onset dementia is confirmed, everyone involved feels an undeniable shift. Intense emotions can run high, and for many, the grieving process starts from the second that the diagnosis is announced. Shock is often the first reaction—this can't be happening, not at this age, not now. Denial might follow, as the reality of the diagnosis can feel too overwhelming to accept. This is exactly what I felt when I first heard my loved one's diagnosis. Mourning is also a common feeling since many people begin to grief the anticipated loss of what was once considered a predictable future—either for themselves or with a beloved member of the family. All of these feelings are natural and valid.

Seeking Support

Navigating this emotional turbulence means that you have to develop a compassionate approach, both towards yourself and those around you. Part of that means allowing yourself to receive support.

Receiving proper support is a must, no matter if you yourself have been diagnosed or if someone close to you has. It can be difficult to handle the strong emotions that come along with a diagnosis all on your own, but seeking support can make the process of moving forward easier. For example, seeking therapeutic support can provide you with a safe space to express and process complex emotions. Therapists who specialize in chronic illness or cognitive disorders can offer you more specific guidance and coping strategies, for example, that respect your feelings while encouraging emotional healing and a future-focused approach to the diagnosis ("Getting Treatment for Depression, Anxiety or Apathy," n.d.).

Also, connecting with peer support groups, whether online or in person, can be incredibly comforting. Sharing your story with others who are on a similar path can reduce the loneliness and isolation that often accompany a dementia diagnosis. Or, if you're a family member to someone with dementia, support groups for loved ones to those with dementia can contribute support, advice, and comfort to your coping toolkit, too. No matter who you are, this journey doesn't have to be walked alone.

Managing Impacts on Family

The impact of an early-onset dementia diagnosis on family dynamics doesn't go unnoticed. For example, it's common that roles within the family shift after a diagnosis has been made. A spouse or a child might take on caregiving responsibilities, drastically shifting the typical family layout that you're used to. For caregivers and those with dementia alike, these changes can be difficult to understand and cope with. To manage the emotions that surround these changes, open communication and emotional resilience are important to think of.

Open communication is crucial in navigating any major family changes. Your family can benefit from discussing feelings, concerns, and the practical aspects of care openly and regularly, ensuring that everyone understands each other and their role in supporting the member with dementia. Communication also includes establishing boundaries and delegating responsibilities fairly to avoid caregiver burnout.

Furthermore, it's important to be resilient. It's easier said than done, I know, but resilience is one of the most important emotional management skills you can develop right now. Emotional resilience refers to our ability to bounce back from setbacks or difficult emotions. It's not a matter of feeling strong all the time but rather developing the ability to recover and adapt in the face of stress and adversity. Cultivating resilience can look like engaging with regular physical activity, keeping up with your hobbies and interests, and working with mental health professionals or your family to determine coping mechanisms.

As you and your family manage the emotions that come along with a dementia diagnosis, remember that the feelings you're experiencing are natural. Throughout this book, we will explore countless strategies for managing life post-diagnosis, leading to better coping and increased comfort wherever possible.

BIOLOGICAL INSIGHTS: HOW EARLY-ONSET DEMENTIA AFFECTS THE BRAIN

In order to understand both the progression of the disease and the symptoms that you or your loved one will experience, you have to first understand the biological changes that occur in the brain due to early-onset dementia.

As dementia develops, the brain experiences significant changes that affect its structure and function. One of the most notable changes is the development of abnormal structures known as plaques and tangles. Plaques are deposits of a protein fragment called beta-amyloid that build up in the spaces between nerve cells. On the other hand, tangles are twisted fibers of another protein called tau that build up inside cells. Though most people develop some plaques and tangles as they age, people with early-onset dementia tend to develop these at a much younger age and at a faster rate, leading to a more rapid decline in brain function ("Inside the Brain," 2020).

These plaques and tangles contribute to the loss of connections between nerve cells and, eventually, the death of these cells and the loss of brain tissue. In younger people, this can be particularly aggressive, affecting multiple components of cognitive function—like memory, reasoning, and emotional regulation. Moreover, the parts of the brain that are responsible for planning and executing complex tasks and behavior are often among the first to be affected ("What Is Dementia?" 2022). This is why symptoms like forgetting important dates, struggling to solve problems, and mood swings are common in people with early-onset dementia and why treatment as early as possible is important. It's also worthwhile to understand that the impact on younger brains can be more life-altering because these individuals are often struck at crucial stages of life—managing careers, families, and active social lives—which demands high cognitive function.

But why does early-onset dementia occur in the first place? Recent research into the causes of early-onset dementia has highlighted a few potential factors that can contribute to the development of the disease ("What Is Dementia? Symptoms, Types, and Diagnosis," 2022):

- **Genetics:** Genetic factors have been explored, and we now know that they can increase the likelihood of someone developing early-onset dementia. If you have a loved one who experienced early-onset dementia, then you're more likely to experience it yourself than someone with no family history of it.
- **Inflammation in the Brain:** Brain inflammation has been linked to early-onset dementia, although more research is needed to understand this link in-depth.
- **Environmental Influences:** Environmental influences like diet have also been shown to play some role in increasing the likelihood of early-onset dementia.

Connecting these biological changes to the symptoms of dementia means that we can understand why dementia manifests in the ways that it does. In turn, we can better tailor interventions to manage symptoms effectively. For example, therapies that focus on cognitive stimulation might be the best to slow the progression of memory loss, while behavioral therapies can help manage changes in personality and mood. Additionally, understanding that these changes are due to the disease and not the person's character can lead to greater empathy and patience among caregivers and family members, improving the quality of care and support provided to individuals with dementia.

DIFFERENTIATING EARLY-ONSET FROM LATER-ONSET DEMENTIA

While both are forms of dementia, it's important to recognize that early-onset and later-onset dementia are different.

Understanding this difference means that you can better advocate for the care of yourself or your loved one based on personalized approaches for the specific diagnosis received.

Clinically and pathologically, these forms of dementia present differently, particularly when it comes to the speed of progression and the nature of cognitive decline. Early-onset dementia typically progresses at a faster rate compared to dementia that occurs later in life. These rapid changes can be challenging to manage since it often results in less time for those with dementia and their families to adapt to each new stage of the disease. Also, the type of cognitive decline can differ. Early-onset dementia often impacts executive functions like problem-solving, organizing, and multitasking, which isn't always the case with later-onset dementia, where memory loss might be more prominent at the outset (Awada 2015).

These differences have a massive impact when it comes to considering the unique struggles of younger people suffering from dementia. People who experience early-onset dementia are usually actively working, raising children, or even caring for their own elderly parents, creating countless complications. Due to these differences, how you and your loved ones manage dementia has to be adapted to fit age-specific needs.

For example, maintaining a job can become difficult as time passes and cognitive abilities decline. This not only affects financial stability but also self-esteem and identity, as work is a major part of how many people define themselves. This might include workplace accommodations, such as adjusting workloads or modifying tasks to match the changing abilities of the person with dementia. In more advanced stages, transitioning from work to retirement can be aided by financial planning services that focus on premature retirement due to disability.

For parents, the challenges of early-onset dementia extend to maintaining parental responsibilities and supporting children through milestones while navigating their own cognitive changes. With knowledge of how early-onset dementia uniquely affects younger people, parenting strategies can be shaped to include more structured routines and possibly involve children appropriately in the care process. The benefits of doing so mean that their children are prepared and supported.

Social engagement also suffers due to declining cognitive skills needed for such interactions, and understanding how to maintain socialization is crucial to feeling fulfilled and happy as the disease progresses. Social strategies, then, might focus on maintaining simpler, more structured social interactions and choosing activities that align with remaining personal strengths.

Michael and Linda: Their Stories

Tailoring an approach for managing dementia always requires personalization. Making an effort to adjust your life to the needs of a diagnosis is always ideal because it allows you to prepare, accommodate, and make transitions more effectively. Michael, unfortunately, was unprepared to handle the challenges of dementia because of its early onset, which caused significant stress for himself and his family. Michael was a former architect and was diagnosed with early-onset Alzheimer's disease at 58 years old. His ability to lead complex projects declined suddenly, forcing him into early retirement. Financially unprepared for this change, Michael and his family faced significant stress, compounded by his increasing need for comprehensive home care.

On the other hand, Linda, diagnosed with Alzheimer's at 72, experienced a slower progression, something that was initially noticed due to her increasing forgetfulness. Her family had more time to plan for her care and adjust to her gradual decline since the later-onset dementia meant slower progression. Through careful planning and the delegation of tasks to members of the family, Linda's family was able to support her with far less stress than Michael's family could support him.

In crafting care plans and support systems for people with early-onset dementia, acknowledging the differences faced as compared to later-onset dementia ensures that interventions are appropriate and effective. It allows for a proactive rather than reactive approach, thus preserving quality of life and independence for as long as possible. As we continue to explore the nuances of early-onset dementia, keeping these distinctions in mind will guide you in providing the most supportive and compassionate care possible.

EARLY SIGNS AND WHEN TO SEEK A PROFESSIONAL OPINION

It can be hard to recognize the early signs of dementia, especially in younger people, where symptoms might be easily dismissed as stress or the byproducts of a busy life. Yet, these initial indicators—subtle as they may be—are vital to understand for early detection and timely intervention.

Signs to Look Out For

When early-onset dementia is a concern, it's helpful to know what signs to look out for. Common signs of early-onset dementia often include (Better Health Channel 2014):

- **Forgetfulness:** While forgetfulness is something we all experience from time to time, early-onset dementia often includes forgetfulness that goes beyond forgetting your keys sometimes. Someone with this disease might experience issues with remembering names, places, or expectations of them to the point that it creates conflict in daily life.
- **Mood Changes:** It's also common for someone with early-onset dementia to experience significant changes in mood. Often, this manifests as being more irritable than normal or becoming easily agitated; however, dramatic bouts of crying and sadness can also occur.
- **Struggling with Common Tasks:** Many people who are experiencing early-onset dementia struggle to manage daily tasks that they were once good at or completed with ease. This can result in frustration, delayed tasks, and more.

These changes can be gradual, almost imperceptible, or they might evolve more rapidly than one might expect. Keeping an eye out for any uncharacteristic behavior—big or small—is a helpful way to spot the signs early.

For younger people, acknowledging that these symptoms could signify something as serious as dementia is often difficult. There is a natural tendency to blame overworking, sleep deprivation, or stress for these symptoms instead. While these are indeed valid reasons for occasional memory lapses or mood swings, when these symptoms persist or worsen, they warrant a closer look. Early recognition is essential to making sure that you or your loved one receive the right support and treatment and that needs, and desires can be accommodated from the beginning of the condition.

When to Seek Help

When these signs begin to interfere with daily life, it is time to seek professional advice. This doesn't mean that help should only be sought out when a person can no longer function; instead, if these signs are causing distress, anxiety, or near-daily difficulties in managing life, help should be sought right away.

The first step in seeking help for early-onset dementia is to visit a primary care physician who can conduct preliminary assessments and rule out other possible causes of the symptoms. As I mentioned earlier, this can include different brain scans and basic tests to make sure that what you're really facing is dementia. Stress, depression, anxiety, and other chronic diseases outside of dementia can cause similar symptoms, and having an accurate diagnosis means having accurate support.

Depending on the findings from that initial visit, the next step may involve consulting specialists such as neurologists or geriatric psychiatrists, who can offer more detailed evaluations and confirm a diagnosis through cognitive tests and neurological examinations. When you reach out to these professionals, it's important to chat with those who have experience with dementia, particularly early-onset types, as they can provide more targeted insights and recommendations. Your general physician can usually offer recommendations for such professionals if you're not sure where to look (Alzheimer's Association 2023).

The Importance of Preparing for Appointments

With that said, prior to visiting the doctor's office, some preparation can be helpful to ensure that all concerns are adequately addressed. Maintaining a symptom diary can be incredibly beneficial; it should include detailed notes on what symptoms have been noticed, their frequency, any patterns that appear relevant, and how they impact daily activities. This record provides healthcare professionals with a clearer picture of what has been happening over time, which can contribute to an accurate diagnosis.

Also, preparing a list of questions to ask during the visit can help make the most of the time spent with the doctor. Questions might include inquiries about the types of diagnostic tests that will be used, the potential causes of the symptoms, the treatment options available, and the implications of the diagnosis on daily life. Don't be afraid to share your concerns or ask for input from a doctor—they're there to help you or your loved one, and no question is a bad question where your health is concerned.

In this context, it becomes clear why understanding and recognizing the early signs of dementia in younger people is so important. It's more than medical treatment—this understanding means that you can adapt to and plan for changes that affect every aspect of life. With appropriate medical advice and support, you can navigate these changes more effectively, maintaining your or your loved one's quality of life and independence for as long as possible. With this understanding in mind, it's time to take advantage of the time you have now to hammer out certain legal considerations.

2

LEGAL AND FINANCIAL PLANNING

It might seem grim to work on legal and financial planning right away—for many people, it can feel like sealing the deal and planning for the end. But take a moment to imagine a day when making choices might not be as straightforward as it is now, where expressing your personal preferences, especially about healthcare, becomes a challenge. It's a situation none of us want to face, but it's a pressing future that those dealing with early-onset dementia have to manage. Planning for legal and financial considerations now means that your future is protected—that your wishes are respected and your comforts solidified.

This chapter is designed to navigate you through setting up a living will and other legal considerations to be your voice when articulating your wishes directly becomes a challenge. Or, if you're reading to help a loved one manage their care, this chapter provides you with everything you need to know to offer your loved one support when it comes to legal and financial planning.

DRAFTING A LIVING WILL: A STEP-BY-STEP GUIDE

The significance of a living will is immense. A living will is a document that outlines your healthcare preferences in different circumstances, covering aspects from the types of medical treatment you wish to receive to your preferences for end-of-life care and pain management. As early-onset dementia progresses, a living will is especially important so that your wishes and decisions are respected when you may be unable to communicate them effectively. A living will speaks for you, providing clear instructions to healthcare providers and relieving your family from the doubt and stress of making these difficult decisions during stressful times.

Components of a Living Will

A living will should clearly outline your healthcare preferences across various scenarios. It typically includes decisions about the use of life-sustaining treatments, such as ventilators and feeding tubes, should you become unable to decide for yourself. It also covers your choices regarding pain management—whether you prefer all available means to alleviate pain or only specific types. Furthermore, your living will should address your wishes concerning end-of-life care, such as hospice care, and the extent of medical intervention you are comfortable with when recovery becomes impossible. Detailing these elements makes sure that your medical care aligns with your values and desires, providing you with dignity and respect in all circumstances (Keene 2022).

Step-by-Step Creation Process

Drafting a living will requires careful consideration and several key steps to ensure it is effective and legally binding:

1. **Talk to a healthcare provider.** First, it is a good idea to consult with a healthcare provider to understand the medical implications of your choices. This conversation equates to personal clarity about the consequences of certain healthcare decisions, helping you make informed choices that truly reflect your wishes.
2. **Consult a legal professional.** Next, consulting a legal professional who specializes in estate planning or elder law is necessary. These professionals can guide you on the legal requirements specific to your state, as the legality of living wills can vary across jurisdictions. It's not enough to write things down on paper and forget about them. An attorney can also help you draft the document to ensure that it is clear, unambiguous, and adheres to all legal standards.
3. **Get your will signed and notarized.** Once drafted, your living will needs to be signed in the presence of witnesses. Depending on your state's laws, these witnesses might need to be non-relatives to avoid potential conflicts of interest down the line. In some cases, the document may also need to be notarized to increase its legal standing.

Review and Updates

Life circumstances and preferences change, and so might your views on medical treatments and end-of-life care. Regularly reviewing your living will while you're able to ensures that it always reflects your latest wishes. It is advisable to review this document at least every few years or after significant life events, such as a new diagnosis, the death of a loved one, or a change in marital status. During the review, you can make amendments as necessary, which should also be done under the guidance of your attorney to ensure that any changes are legally sound. This way, you don't have to worry about being trapped with the decisions you made when first diagnosed if those aren't what you want later in life.

Values Journaling Prompt

Take some time to reflect on what values are most important to you in terms of medical care. What matters most to you if you are unable to make decisions for yourself? Reflecting on these questions can help clarify your thoughts before you begin drafting your living will. Write these reflections down—they can be a useful reference when discussing your wishes with your lawyer and family.

In crafting your living will, you are taking a proactive step toward managing your future and looking out for yourself down the line. Crafting a living will means preserving your peace of mind and making care easier for your loved ones.

UNDERSTANDING AND SETTING UP DURABLE POWER OF ATTORNEY

Another crucial step to be taken when it comes to future-focused planning is setting up a durable power of attorney (DPOA). Setting up a DPOA must be done while you are still capable, and it allows you to appoint someone you trust to manage your financial and legal affairs if there comes a time when you are no longer able to do so yourself. The term "durable" refers to the DPOA's ability to remain in effect even after you, the principal, become unable to make decisions or changes of your own accord.

The role of a durable power of attorney in the context of dementia is significant. We can't always account for every situation that might arise when setting up a living will, and a DPOA covers those gaps. Your DPOA will have the ability to manage both major considerations and daily interactions (i.e., paying your bills) so that you're always taken care of. The appointed person acts as a decision-maker according to your wishes and best interests, so it's important to pick the right person ("Frequently Asked Questions about Durable Powers of Attorney for Health Care," n.d.).

Selecting an Attorney-in-Fact

Picking the right person to act as your attorney-in-fact (the person you pick to carry out your DPOA requests) requires thoughtful consideration. Someone who makes a great attorney-in-fact will be trustworthy, financially astute, well-organized, and, ideally, will have a good understanding of your personal values and desires. This person could be a family member, a close friend, or even a professional such as an accountant or lawyer. The key is their ability to handle responsibility with integrity and their commitment to acting in your best interests, keeping in mind the legal and ethical obligations that come with the role. This means that emotional stability is also crucial, and a willingness to be unbiased even in stressful situations is also vital (Gordon 2024).

Granting Power of Attorney

Just like setting up a living will, the legal process to grant power of attorney involves several important steps and varies by jurisdiction. Generally, you will start with drafting the power of attorney document, which clearly outlines the scope of authority granted to the attorney-in-fact. This document should be as specific as possible to avoid any ambiguity about what powers are being delegated; in other words, it needs to be clear what your attorney-in-fact can and cannot do. Common powers granted include handling financial transactions, managing real estate assets, and making healthcare decisions, among others.

Once the document is drafted, you have to sign it while at least two adult witnesses who are not the attorney-in-fact are present. Some states also require the document to be notarized. After the signing, the document should be stored in a secure yet accessible place, and copies should be given to the attorney-in-fact, your financial institutions, and perhaps your doctor to ensure that it can be easily referenced by all parties involved in your care when needed ("Finalizing Your Durable Power of Attorney for Finances" n.d.).

FINANCIAL PLANNING STRATEGIES FOR EARLY-ONSET DEMENTIA

As you adapt to living with early-onset dementia, it's also necessary to think about financial planning, both for the safety of your current needs and for the security of your future care. Budgeting for future care involves more than just tallying monthly expenses—it also includes anticipating costs that are likely to arise due to your condition, as well as ensuring that funds are available to maintain a comfortable quality of life as your needs evolve. Medical expenses, in-home care services, and potentially long-term care facilities are significant costs that should be factored into your financial planning from as early on as possible. Moreover, early and accurate budgeting helps in setting realistic expectations and provides a clearer picture, which is essential for peace of mind for both you and your loved ones.

To start, it's a good idea to look at your current medical expenses. If you have current medical expenses related to managing your dementia, you can project these costs into the future, considering the likely progression of your condition. This is a great way to start with an estimate of how much you might need. If you're entirely unsure of how much you might need, then a financial advisor who specializes in medical concerns can offer support that leads you to a financially secure future.

Also, as you plan, don't forget to include potential increases in costs due to changing health needs. It's common for treatment needs to become more severe with age, and in order to keep up with those costs, your financial planning needs to account for that. You also have to account for medical expenses adjacent to the care itself, like transportation to appointments, home modifications or equipment, etc. Similarly, if in-home care or eventual transition to a care facility is something you expect to need or use, researching current rates for these services and accounting for annual increases can help in creating a more accurate budget.

Then, there are investments to consider. For many people, investment goes hand-in-hand when it comes to end-of-life financial management. In fact, investment is often recommended as a strategy for retirement, so there's no reason it can't be a strategy for affording long-term medical care as well. If you haven't already, this is a good time to consider setting up an investment account specifically earmarked for future care-related concerns. Diversifying the investments tied to this account can help manage risk and increase potential returns.

Government aid and support programs are another key player in alleviating the financial burdens associated with early-onset dementia. For instance, Medicaid provides health coverage to millions of Americans, including eligible low-income adults, children, pregnant women, elderly adults, and people with disabilities Medicaid programs can help cover costs like nursing home care and personal care services, which are often necessary as dementia progresses. Likewise, if you have worked long enough and paid Social Security taxes, Social Security Disability Insurance (SSDI) may be available to you. This can be a big help when it comes to replacing some of your income if you are unable to work due to your health condition. It is beneficial to investigate these options early on, as applications and approvals can take considerable time—even up to a year in some cases ("Medicare Enrollment Numbers," 2023).

NAVIGATING INSURANCE AND BENEFITS FOR YOUNGER PATIENTS

Understanding the world of insurance and benefits can feel overwhelming, especially when you're already dealing with the complexities of early-onset dementia. Knowing which options are right for you might seem daunting, but ultimately, it's an invaluable aspect of caring for your health throughout the progress of your condition. It's important that you feel empowered to manage insurance and benefits effectively in order to maximize such benefits while reducing the associated stress.

Understanding Insurance Options

Health insurance is your first line of defense. Most plans typically cover visits to your doctor, hospital stays, and medications, all of which are necessary for managing dementia. However, with early-onset dementia, you might also need to consider the benefits of long-term care insurance. This type of insurance is specifically designed to cover services that regular health insurance doesn't, such as assistance with daily living activities and nursing home care. You might also consider disability insurance, which provides income replacement if you are no longer able to work due to your disability.

To maximize your insurance benefits, start by thoroughly understanding your policy details—know what each policy covers and what it doesn't. For health insurance, understand your deductible, out-of-pocket maximum, and what services are covered under your plan. For long-term care insurance, get a clear idea of the conditions under which you can claim benefits, the duration of coverage, and the daily or monthly benefit amounts. Finally, with disability insurance, understand the definition of disability used, the waiting period before benefits start, and the duration of coverage. If this information feels dense or confusing, you can always consult with an insurance specialist who can explain these details in clear, simple terms and help you plan accordingly ("Does Long-Term Care Insurance Cover Memory Care? A Comprehensive Guide" 2023).

Dealing With Challenges

Sometimes, insurance is a bit finicky; there are challenges that you have to know how to mitigate for proper coverage and care planning. That said, dealing with insurance companies can sometimes be challenging, especially when a claim is denied. If you find yourself in this situation, start by understanding why the claim was denied—the reason should be stated in the denial letter. If the denial is due to missing information or a misunderstanding about your coverage, submitting an appeal with the necessary documentation might resolve the issue. This is why you should keep detailed records of all your medical appointments, prescriptions, and any communications with your insurance company, as these documents can save the day when you need to support your case.

LEGAL AND FINANCIAL PLANNING | 37

But what if your insurance coverage is just insufficient when it comes to covering your healthcare needs? This is when it's a good time to explore alternative coverage options. Supplemental policies, such as Medigap, can help cover costs that your regular health insurance does not, like copayments, deductibles, and coinsurance. Also, take some time to look into community health programs that offer services based on sliding scale fees or that are funded by local government or charitable organizations. These programs can provide valuable support ("What's Medicare Supplement Insurance (Medigap)? | Medicare," n.d.).

PROTECTING ASSETS AND PLANNING FOR LONG-TERM CARE NEEDS

Navigating early-onset dementia also involves considerations relating to the protection of your assets. Asset protection strategies ensure that your resources are preserved to provide for your care and support without being excessively depleted through healthcare and living expenses. Setting up trusts is a commonly employed method. When you place assets in a trust, you control how your assets are used after your ability to make financial decisions may diminish. Trusts can be designed to distribute funds in specific ways, ensuring that they are used for your care and benefit over time, according to the terms you set.

Another option that you have is transferring assets for protection, which needs careful handling to avoid future legal complications or penalties. I highly recommend that you consult with a legal advisor who specializes in elder law to navigate these transfers properly. They can help structure the transfers to minimize any potential penalties or issues with benefit eligibility. This is where understanding the legal structures that can safeguard your assets becomes incredibly valuable. For example, an irrevocable trust can provide asset protection because once established, the terms cannot easily be changed, and assets placed within the trust are typically not considered personal assets susceptible to claims by creditors.

As you consider these options, it is equally important to plan comprehensively for long-term care. This includes evaluating potential care facilities well in advance and understanding the specific services they offer, as well as their costs. Knowing what type of care facility—be it assisted living, a nursing home, or specialized dementia care—is appropriate for your situation helps in making an informed decision. Moreover, planning for possible relocation early on gives you the time to visit and evaluate various facilities, assess their quality of care, and their ability to meet your future needs. This ensures that you find a place that feels right and can help ease the transition when the time comes.

As you move forward, remember that protecting your future through a living will, power of attorney, and financial considerations is essential in making sure that your care represents your wishes. These steps allow you to have a say in your future care, even when you might not be able to communicate your desires on your own.

3

DAILY LIFE ADJUSTMENTS

Now that we have legal concerns out of the way, we have to talk about your environment and daily life. Dementia can be disarming and scary, and having an environment that is comforting and accessible is a must. Different parts of the environment that we ignore today, like patterned carpets and crooked furniture, easily become obstacles and challenges for those suffering from dementia. As you explore this chapter, you will master key considerations in adjusting your environment and daily life to fit the needs of yourself—or your loved one with dementia.

MODIFYING YOUR HOME FOR SAFETY AND ACCESSIBILITY

Creating a safe and accessible home environment is fundamental for anyone living with early-onset dementia. It involves carefully assessing your living space to identify and mitigate potential hazards, as well as thoughtful modifications to enhance both safety and comfort. Let's explore how you can assess your home for safety, implement necessary modifications, and arrange your living space in a way that supports both independence and well-being.

Assessing Home Safety

Begin with a thorough walk-through of your home to assess its general safety, including any places that need to be modified for safety. Look for hazards such as poor lighting, loose rugs, cluttered walkways, and any obstacles that could pose a risk for trips and falls. Check that all areas of your home are well-lit, especially places like stairways, hallways, and bathrooms. Lighting is important for visibility and comfort and can also be used as a cue for yourself or a loved one who might forget where certain rooms are. Additionally, ensure that safety devices such as smoke detectors and carbon monoxide alarms are in working order and placed appropriately throughout the home.

Adaptive Modifications

Once you've ensured that the basics are ready to go, safety modifications should be the next consideration. These changes might include:

- installing grab bars in the bathroom near the toilet and shower, which can provide stability and support
- placing non-slip mats in the shower, bath, and other slippery surfaces to prevent falls, one of the most common accidents that can have serious consequences for someone with balance or mobility issues

DAILY LIFE ADJUSTMENTS | 41

- removing or securing loose rugs and carpets or replacing them with anti-slip versions to ensure safer movement around the house
- adding handrails on both sides of any staircases for added safety, and if possible, a stairlift to facilitate movement between floors ("Home Safety" 2021)

Creating a Dementia-Friendly Layout

Arranging your home to minimize confusion and maximize ease of movement facilitates safety and accessibility, too. This process involves more than just decluttering. For example, creating a clear path of movement throughout your home and organizing each space logically and simply can help prevent confusion and maximize independence as dementia progresses. It's also a good idea to keep frequently used items in easy-to-remember places and to consider labeling cabinets and drawers with words or pictures that describe their contents. This can help reduce the frustration associated with memory lapses.

Use of Safety Technologies

Incorporating technology can significantly enhance the safety of a home for someone with dementia. It can be helpful, for example, to install automatic shut-off devices on appliances like stoves and irons to prevent accidents if they are accidentally left on. Also, automated sensors can be placed on doors and windows to alert caregivers if they are opened, which is particularly useful for preventing wandering, a common and dangerous issue in the later stages of dementia. Similarly, the use of motion sensor lights that automatically illuminate when movement is detected can improve safety.

Throughout these adjustments, it's important to maintain a balance between safety and maintaining a homely atmosphere. Changes should enhance safety without making the home feel less comforting or more clinical so that you or your loved one still feels comfortable and at ease at home (van Dyk and Dono 2017).

EFFECTIVE COMMUNICATION STRATEGIES AS DEMENTIA PROGRESSES

As dementia progresses, the ways in which you might experience and interact with the world change, particularly in how you communicate. Understanding these changes is important for maintaining relationships and ensuring that your needs are met. Dementia can notably affect your ability to find the right words, follow conversations, and express thoughts coherently as a result of changes in the brain areas responsible for language and information processing. Recognizing what to expect as these changes unfold can help you and your loved ones adapt more effectively to these evolving communication needs.

One of the most noticeable changes in communication for someone with dementia is the increasing difficulty in finding the right words. This can lead to pauses in speech as your loved one searches for what they want to say, which might cause frustration or withdrawal from conversations. Moreover, they might find it hard to follow complex sentences or rapidly shifting topics, making it challenging to keep up with group discussions or fast-paced dialogues. As a response, adapting the way conversations are held can significantly benefit your engagement and understanding of your loved one. For instance, you can make a conscious effort to use simpler words and shorter sentences when speaking to your loved one. This clarity helps in reducing cognitive load, allowing them to process information more comfortably. Additionally, maintaining a calm and clear tone of voice can make a big difference; a direct and gentle tone does a lot for minimizing misunderstandings and enhancing their ability to follow along.

Non-verbal cues like body language, facial expressions, and touch play a major role in conveying messages and emotions. For someone with dementia, these non-verbal forms of communication become extremely important. A smile, a reassuring touch, or a calm demeanor can communicate safety and affection, helping to bridge gaps where words fall short. Encouraging those around you to be expressive in their gestures and to use physical contact, like holding hands, can improve the quality of connections and provide comfort. If you're reading this as a caregiver, I encourage you to make an effort to communicate non-verbally in a gentle, caring manner.

Creating an environment conducive to effective communication is equally important. This means minimizing distractions that can make conversations and understanding more difficult. Reducing background noise by turning off the television or moving to a quieter space, for example, can help you focus on the conversation at hand. Visual distractions can be minimized. Also, maintaining eye contact and ensuring the room is well-lit may make it easier for you to see facial expressions and lip movements.

Understanding and adjusting to communication challenges presented by dementia is critical for your loved one—it helps them continue to have fulfilling conversations and interactions. Dementia is often very isolating to deal with, which means that managing communication-related concerns is a part of shifting daily life to accommodate your diagnosis in a meaningful way. The effort of shifting methods of communication is well-worth the payoff of happy conversations and fulfilling engagement.

MANAGING WORK-LIFE AFTER DIAGNOSIS

As mentioned earlier, navigating the workplace after a diagnosis presents unique challenges and requires careful consideration, especially when deciding whether you want to disclose your condition to your employer and colleagues. This decision is deeply personal and can definitely impact your professional life. On one hand, sharing your diagnosis can result in greater understanding and support at work. It can facilitate access to necessary accommodations that can help maintain your productivity and job satisfaction; for instance, your boss might better understand why you might need a flexible schedule or adjustments to your workload. On the other hand, there is the risk of stigma, potential discrimination, and even jeopardizing your career progression. Some might view the diagnosis as a decline in your professional capability, which could influence their decisions on your responsibilities or the future within the company.

Disclosing Your Diagnosis and Accommodations

If you choose to disclose your diagnosis, it is important to carefully plan how you will approach this conversation. It might be helpful to start by speaking with a human resources (HR) professional who can guide you on the best practices and legal protections under disability laws, such as the Americans with Disabilities Act (ADA) if you are in the United States. These laws are designed to protect you from discrimination and ensure that you have access to reasonable accommodations that can help you perform your job effectively (U.S. Department Of Labor 2024). When discussing your diagnosis, be clear about the specific support or changes you need to continue working effectively so that your employer can meet those needs. It's also helpful to emphasize your commitment to your role and discuss ways you can maintain your performance, possibly including adjustments to your responsibilities or working hours, so that your employer understands your dedication.

On the subject of workplace accommodations, having those accommodations in place can be significant in helping you manage your job duties while dealing with symptoms of dementia. Possible accommodations that you can ask for include a quieter workspace to reduce distractions, flexible work hours to manage fatigue, or the possibility to work from home as needed. Technology can also be a wonderful aid. Using software that helps organize tasks or setting up reminders for important deadlines, for instance, can help you keep track of tasks. It may also be useful to reduce your workload or delegate certain responsibilities that have become challenging, allowing you to focus on areas where you can still perform strongly.

Establishing a support network within your workplace is just as important. Your support network can include colleagues who understand your condition and can provide daily support and encouragement. It's helpful to identify allies in the workplace who can help facilitate this support system, whether it's through regular check-ins, assistance with tasks, or simply providing companionship and understanding. Additionally, staying connected with the HR department can ensure you have continuous access to resources and support that can aid in managing your work life. HR can even help mediate any issues that arise with colleagues or supervisors as a result of your condition, ensuring that your work environment remains supportive and respectful.

Workplace Transitional Considerations

There's the matter of planning for a transition from work to retirement or part-time employment to consider as well. This transition requires careful financial planning to ensure that you can maintain your livelihood. Before quitting your job or making changes to your employment, make it a point to consult with financial advisors who specialize in retirement planning, particularly under circumstances involving health-related work exits. They can provide guidance on managing your retirement savings, accessing disability benefits, and restructuring investments to support your financial needs long-term. It's also wise to discuss these plans with your family and any other advisors to ensure that all aspects of your transition, including health insurance and other benefits, are well managed.

Navigating your professional life after an early-onset dementia diagnosis isn't easy, but with the right considerations and planning, as outlined above, it doesn't have to be a challenge either. Managing how you disclose your condition, the accommodations you request, and other work-related affairs means preserving your career and overall well-being as you manage dementia and its difficulties.

NUTRITION AND PHYSICAL HEALTH: BEST PRACTICES

As you make shifts in your lifestyle, nutritional considerations are helpful for managing symptoms. Studies show that nutrition can have a positive impact on preserving cognitive functions, lifting mood, and reducing the speed of progression ("What Do We Know about Diet and Prevention of Alzheimer's Disease?" n.d.). Therefore, making positive nutritional changes can support your well-being, and there are a few changes that you can consider.

Nutrient Considerations

Foods rich in omega-3 fatty acids, such as salmon, flaxseeds, and walnuts, are renowned for their brain-boosting properties (Dighriri et al., 2022). These nutrients support the building of new neural connections and the maintenance of existing cellular structures in the brain. Similarly, antioxidants found abundantly in berries, leafy greens, and nuts combat oxidative stress—a contributor to brain aging and dementia ("Diet and Dementia | Alzheimer's Society"). Incorporating these foods into your daily meals can provide your brain with the nutrients it needs to function optimally.

Furthermore, whole grains, lean proteins, and a variety of fruits and vegetables should form the basis of your diet. These foods offer a wide range of essential nutrients that help maintain overall physical health, which is instrumental in managing dementia symptoms. Different diets can incorporate these nutrients effectively for easy nutritional management. The Mediterranean diet, for example, which emphasizes these food groups, has been associated with a lower risk of cognitive decline ("MIND and Mediterranean Diets Linked to Fewer Signs of Alzheimer's Brain Pathology," 2023).

Hydration is often overlooked when thinking about nutrition, but it's another pressing aspect of your health that requires attention ("6 Dehydration Facts That May Surprise You," n.d.). As you age, your body's ability to conserve water decreases, and you might lose the ability to know when you're thirsty as easily—which can quickly lead to dehydration. This is especially concerning with dementia, where the usual cues to drink water might go unnoticed. Dehydration can exacerbate confusion and lead to further decline in cognitive function, which is why it is essential to actively manage your fluid intake (Fayaz 2016). Setting regular reminders to drink water, keeping a water bottle within easy reach, and incorporating hydrating foods like cucumbers, melons, and soups into your diet are all great strategies to maintain adequate hydration. Moreover, encouraging the consumption of fluids throughout the day, rather than relying on the sensation of thirst, can prevent dehydration and the risks it creates.

Mealtime Concerns

Mealtime presents its own set of challenges as dementia progresses. You might face issues like decreased appetite, forgetting to eat, and difficulties using eating utensils, all of which can interfere with your ability to eat enough nutritional food each day. There are a few techniques that you can implement as someone with dementia or a caregiver to make these concerns less pressing. For instance:

- creating a pleasant and relaxing mealtime environment can help stimulate appetite and make eating more enjoyable.
- using adaptive utensils designed for easier handling can assist you if you struggle with coordination or grip.
- plates with high-contrast colors can also make it easier for you to distinguish food, which can help increase food intake.
- smaller, more frequent meals might be more manageable and less overwhelming than three large meals, especially if your appetite is reduced.

Each meal is an opportunity to consume nourishing foods that support brain health and physical well-being, making it vital to adapt these strategies to fit your changing needs. Eating well means that you can potentially delay the progression of dementia, which is certainly desirable.

Exercise and Physical Activity

As you make strides to take care of your physical health post-diagnosis, physical activity cannot be ignored. Regular exercise not only benefits your cardiovascular health but also has a direct impact on brain function ("Exercise Can Boost Your Memory and Thinking Skills," 2023). Activities that increase your heart rate, such as walking, cycling, or swimming, enhance blood flow to the brain and can improve neural connections. Beyond that, strength training, even with light weights or body-weight exercises, helps maintain muscle mass and supports overall mobility and balance, reducing the risk of falls. Even exercises like yoga and tai chi can improve both physical balance and mental focus, contributing to better cognitive health. It is important to find activities that you enjoy and can participate in regularly. The goal is to integrate physical activity into your daily routine in a way that feels rewarding and feasible, leading both to enjoyment and long-term health benefits.

Incorporating these best practices into your daily life requires commitment and adaptation, but the benefits they bring in managing dementia are substantial. By focusing on a diet rich in brain-healthy nutrients, ensuring regular hydration, adapting mealtime strategies to meet changing needs, and maintaining an active lifestyle, you create a robust framework for supporting both your cognitive and physical health as you navigate life with early-onset dementia. These adjustments not only enhance your ability to manage the symptoms of dementia but also significantly improve your overall quality of life, allowing you to engage more fully with the world around you.

TECHNOLOGY AND TOOLS TO SUPPORT INDEPENDENCE

Embracing technology as a part of your daily life can significantly enhance your ability to manage daily life with early-onset dementia. Technology designed for accessibility and to ease symptoms of dementia in specific have the ability to promote independence while ensuring your safety and comfort. A variety of assistive devices and software solutions are specifically designed to support people with conditions like dementia, which means that they can easily be implemented to help you maintain your autonomy and reduce reliance on caregivers for everyday tasks.

Assistive Technology Devices

Innovations in assistive technology offer practical solutions that can help you manage aspects of your daily routine more independently. Automated medication dispensers are one example of such tools. These dispensers are designed to alleviate the burden of remembering medication schedules. They can be programmed to dispense the right amount of medication at specified times, and they often come with alarms or reminders to take your medicine. This ensures that you stay on top of your medication regimen and the risk of accidental overdose or missed doses, which can be common as a result of memory challenges.

Another great tool for enhancing safety and independence is GPS trackers. Wearable GPS devices can help reduce wandering, a common and concerning issue for those with dementia. These trackers can alert caregivers if you wander outside of a predefined safe zone so that they can locate you quickly and keep you safe. If you're a caregiver yourself, devices like these can make it so that you never have to worry about your loved one getting lost or wandering off when you're busy or otherwise unable to be present.

You can even find simplified appliances, such as microwaves with preset buttons and simplified interfaces. As dementia progresses, it can often be daunting to use technology on your own, even if you were previously familiar with a device. The low confidence or confusion that you face can make it hard to feel comfortable preparing your own food, but devices like these make cooking safer and easier by reducing the complexity and steps involved in operating conventional appliances ("7 Dementia Friendly Kitchen Appliances & Devices " 2022).

Apps and Software

Did you know that there are several apps and software programs specifically tailored to meet the needs of individuals with dementia? These wonderful tools can help you manage daily tasks, keep track of appointments, and stay connected with loved people. Memory aid apps, for instance, can help you store important information such as names, faces, and important dates, which can be easily retrieved to aid memory. Beyond that, daily planning apps can help with organizing your day by providing reminders for appointments, meals, and other necessary activities. If you implement apps and software like these, it means that even on more challenging days, you have the support you need to manage your schedule effectively (Desai 2024).

Home Automation

You can also automate parts of your home to increase accessibility. Smart home technologies can transform your living environment into a safer, more comfortable, and more manageable space. Systems that allow you to control lighting, temperature, and security devices from a single, simplified interface can significantly improve your ability to manage your household independently, especially when technology begins to seem too confusing. For example, automated lighting systems can be programmed to adjust based on the time of day or activated by motion sensors, reducing the risk of accidents caused by poor lighting while improving your sense of time. Similarly, smart thermostats can ensure that your home remains at a comfortable temperature without the need for manual adjustments, which can sometimes be forgotten or be physically challenging (Lennon n.d.).

Accessibility and Usability

When choosing technology to support you or your loved one's independence, make sure that you consider the accessibility and usability of each device or app. Look for solutions that are specifically designed with ease of use in mind, ideally requiring minimal steps to operate. Large buttons, clear displays, and voice-activated features can make technological devices more accessible if you face challenges with dexterity or vision. Additionally, choosing products that offer robust customer support and user guides can help ensure that you get the most out of your technology without feeling overwhelmed.

As this chapter concludes, remember that each piece of technology or technique you integrate into your life is more than adhering to a recommendation; it's part of a powerful motion toward maintaining your autonomy and enhancing your quality of life. From ensuring that your physical health is maintained to simplifying daily tasks through smart home devices, these considerations empower you to manage your daily life with greater ease and confidence. As we move forward, the next chapter will build on the foundation we've established here, exploring strategies for maintaining healthy levels of emotional and psychological support as you navigate dementia.

4

EMOTIONAL AND PSYCHOLOGICAL SUPPORT

When the reality of an early-onset dementia diagnosis settles in, it's not just the mind that feels the shock but also the heart. Emotions can swing wildly from disbelief and anger to profound sadness in an instant. It's a sign of the deeply personal and all-encompassing impact this diagnosis has on your life. You might find yourself mourning the future you envisioned, grappling with uncertainty, or feeling isolated in your experiences. This emotional journey is profound, complex, and deeply unique for each person. That said, embracing and understanding these emotions, as well as learning to navigate them, means that you can find a path through the turmoil that leads to a place of greater peace and resilience.

DEALING WITH GRIEF AND EMOTIONAL TURMOIL POST-DIAGNOSIS

Understanding the Grieving Process

The grief that accompanies a diagnosis of early-onset dementia can be multifaceted, involving layers of loss that extend beyond simply feeling shocked. Elisabeth Kübler-Ross's model of the five stages of grief—denial, anger, bargaining, depression, and acceptance—offers a framework that many people find helpful (Tyrrell et al., 2023). While these stages offer a lot of insight when it comes to understanding grief, they also aren't linear and may not occur in any specific order. You might find yourself oscillating between feelings of anger and moments of acceptance, or you might experience waves of depression before feeling ready to confront the reality of the diagnosis. Understanding that these emotional responses are normal can help you give yourself the grace to experience and express these feelings without judgment.

Personal Coping Strategies

Working through your emotional responses requires tools that align with your personal experience and preferences. Journaling, for example, offers a private space to express your thoughts and emotions—serving as a reflective outlet where you can pour out your fears, frustrations, and hopes. Keeping a journal that allows you to reflect can be helpful for dealing with anxieties, anger, and concerns without worrying about how others might think of you, which improves your ability to manage those emotions.

Mindfulness exercises, such as meditation or focused breathing, can be a part of your coping toolkit as well. These exercises can help manage anxiety and stress by anchoring you in the present moment, often providing a calming effect. Even meditating or otherwise engaging in mindfulness for ten minutes a day can improve your emotional regulation and help you work through the grief accompanying you or your loved one's diagnosis. And, if you're a caregiver, helping your loved one work with mindfulness can present an opportunity for bonding while soothing their mind.

I always recommend engaging in hobbies or activities that you love—be it painting, gardening, or listening to music—for emotional relief. As my family supported my loved one through dementia, each of us made time to engage in our personal hobbies for coping, including my loved one, who was diagnosed. These activities brought us joy and a sense of normalcy amidst the chaos, which is why I highly recommend carving this time out for anyone involved in managing dementia.

Family Dynamics and Grief

The loved ones who surround someone diagnosed with dementia—be it you or a different member of your family—are likely navigating their own grief and may experience emotions differently based on their relationship to the person with dementia and their role in caregiving. A dementia diagnosis can create widespread grief and shift family dynamics;

family members have to be willing to communicate openly about these emotions—and to offer support and understanding to each other. Creating a family ritual, such as weekly dinners or regular family meetings, can provide a consistent space for everyone to check in and share their feelings and experiences. These gatherings can strengthen family bonds and provide mutual support, making the emotional journey less isolating for everyone involved.

Seeking Professional Help

Sometimes, emotions can become overwhelming, and the support from family or friends might not be enough. If this sounds like your experience, it can be deeply helpful to seek professional support. Therapists or counselors who specialize in chronic illnesses or dementia can offer more targeted strategies to cope with the emotional challenges posed by dementia. As mentioned earlier, they also provide a safe space to explore your feelings and can help you develop coping strategies or an understanding that is tailored to your situation. Therapy can be beneficial for anyone involved—including caregivers and extended family.

Coping Strategies Journaling Prompt

Take a moment to reflect on your emotional journey since you found out about the diagnosis. What feelings have been the most challenging for you? How have you attempted to cope with these emotions? Writing down your thoughts can help you understand your emotional patterns and identify what coping strategies have been most effective or where you might need additional support.

In navigating the emotional aftermath of an early-onset dementia diagnosis, understanding and acknowledging your feelings are the first steps toward healing. Utilizing personal coping strategies, fostering open communication with family, and seeking professional help when needed are all ways that you can manage the emotional challenges of dementia with strength and resilience.

SUPPORT SYSTEMS: BUILDING AND MAINTAINING RELATIONSHIPS

If you or a loved one have dementia, there's no way around it: You need a support system. A support system is a group of people who are willing to help when you're experiencing a hard time, either by offering support, advice, or something else. This system should ideally contain a broad spectrum of relationships and resources, including family, friends, healthcare providers, and community connections. These networks play an invaluable role in providing practical help, emotional support, and valuable information that can make managing everyday life with dementia more manageable.

Identifying Supportive People

The first step towards building this support system is to identify who in your circle can be part of this network. Family and close friends are often the primary sources of support. Still, it's also important to include professionals such as your doctors, nurses, or a social worker who understand your medical needs and can offer specialized guidance. Beyond this immediate circle, community resources such as local dementia support groups, community centers offering activities for those with cognitive impairments, and online forums can widen this network, providing both you and your caregivers with additional layers of support.

Maintaining Supportive Relationships

Maintaining the relationships that you have with your support system requires open communication about your needs and the impact of dementia on your life. Regular check-ins with family and friends can keep them informed about your condition and any changes in your needs or abilities. These check-ins also provide an opportunity for you to express your emotional state, discuss any challenges you're facing, and receive reassurance and support. In terms of professional relationships, keeping regular appointments and being honest about your symptoms can help your healthcare providers give you the best care possible. It's also beneficial to have a family member or friend attend these appointments with you to ensure all information is understood and retained.

Community Engagement

Community engagement is a great way to ensure emotional health while expanding your support network. If you feel comfortable doing so, participating in community events, joining clubs or groups that interest you, or even attending local gatherings can provide a sense of normalcy and continuity in your life. These activities not only stimulate your mind and keep you active but also help in sustaining a social identity beyond your diagnosis. They offer the chance to meet others who might be navigating similar paths, which leads to opportunities to share experiences and learn from each other in supportive environments.

Digital Engagement

The rise of digital platforms has significantly enhanced the accessibility of support for those who face mobility challenges or live in areas with fewer resources. It can be hard to leave the home or access communities for many people with dementia, but online forums and social media groups dedicated to dementia support can change the game. These platforms allow you to connect with a global community of people who understand your experiences and can offer real-time support and advice. Virtual support groups, webinars on managing dementia, chatrooms, and online recreational activities tailored to your interests and abilities can all be accessed from the comfort of your home so that you can remain connected and supported regardless of physical limitations like limited mobility (Anderson et al. 2022).

In building and sustaining these support networks, the focus should always be on creating meaningful interactions that reinforce your sense of value and belonging. Creating relationships that are socially meaningful and supportive of your well-being can be improved when you take the time to learn about how to find, maintain, and improve those connections.

TECHNIQUES FOR MANAGING CAREGIVER STRESS AND AVOIDING BURNOUT

If you're a caregiver, then this section is for you. And if you have dementia, please never feel ashamed that your caregiver experiences hardship—it's not your fault and is the natural result of changing lifestyles so rapidly. Your caregiver loves and wants to support you deeply, but that requires them to support themselves, too. Caregiver burnout is never something you should worry about as someone with dementia.

That said, as a caregiver, you are undertaking a commitment of love and support for someone—and that commitment requires emotional, physical, and psychological stamina. As a caregiver, you might find yourself facing a multitude of responsibilities that can, over time, lead to significant stress and even burnout. You have to be able to recognize the signs of caregiver stress early, which can manifest in various forms, including irritability, sleep disturbances, physical fatigue, and feelings of despair or helplessness. These symptoms might creep up subtly, which is why it is vital for you to stay attuned to your own well-being as you care for your loved one. For instance, you may notice that your patience wears thin more quickly or that you feel exhausted despite adequate rest, signaling that it's time to reassess your routine and incorporate more self-care. Addressing stress and caregiver burnout right away is necessary to keep yourself healthy and remain vigilant to the needs of your loved one.

Managing Stress

All caregivers experience stress at one point or another. Managing that stress effectively involves a combination of personal strategies and external support. When you constantly have to be attentive to support someone else, it can be helpful to have several relaxation techniques on hand that are quick and easy yet impactful. For example, techniques such as guided imagery, deep breathing exercises, or meditation can significantly reduce stress levels and enhance your ability to respond to daily challenges with a clearer mind.

Another option that you have is structured respite care, where you take deliberate breaks from caregiving. Whether it's a few hours each week or a longer period facilitated by family, friends, or professional services, you should always feel comfortable taking time to step away, which can help you recharge and maintain your health. Respite services are safe and often affordable, so they can provide you with an accessible way to take a break and recharge.

Self-Care for Caregivers

Of course, we can't forget about self-care. Regular physical activity, sufficient sleep, and proper nutrition are necessary practices that positively impact your capacity to manage stress and remain resilient. Physical activity, in particular, can help with both reducing stress and improving overall health. Even simple activities like walking or gentle stretching can make a difference. Prioritizing sleep is equally important; getting poor sleep or not enough rest can impair your ability to think clearly and manage emotions effectively, which are needed in caregiving. And just like a diet rich in fruits, vegetables, lean proteins, and whole grains is good for your loved one with dementia, it's good for you, too! Eating well provides the energy you need to handle the demands of caregiving.

Seeking Professional Support as a Caregiver

Professional support for caregivers is an invaluable option. It's completely normal to feel like you need support as a caregiver—it's no small task. Meeting with a counselor or taking advantage of caregiver support programs can grant you the strategies needed to manage stress and cope with the emotional demands of caregiving. These professionals can offer personalized advice and support that makes it easier for you to navigate the complexities of caregiving with more confidence and less strain. Additionally, caregiver training programs can equip you with practical skills and knowledge about dementia to enhance your caregiving capabilities and reduce anxiety about how to handle various aspects of care. These programs often also offer opportunities to connect with other caregivers, creating a community of support and shared understanding ("Educational Programs and Dementia Care Resources" 2021).

COUNSELING AND THERAPY OPTIONS FOR FAMILIES

When a family member is diagnosed with early-onset dementia, the ripple effects touch every aspect of family life. Such a significant change has the power to alter relationships and daily dynamics in quite striking ways. In times like these, therapy can be a powerful resource that guides your family through the uncertainties, emotional stress, and relational adjustments of a dementia diagnosis. Various therapeutic approaches offer pathways to understanding and managing the emotional and psychological challenges that arise.

Cognitive Behavioral Therapy (CBT)

Cognitive behavioral therapy (CBT) is particularly effective in helping individuals and families develop coping strategies to deal with the behavioral changes that dementia can bring. CBT focuses on the interactions between thoughts, feelings, and behaviors and can, therefore, help family members adjust their expectations and reactions. As a result, it then becomes easier for families to maintain a positive home environment.

Grief Counseling

Grief counseling is another form of therapy that caregivers and loved ones related to someone with dementia can access. It might feel odd to seek grief counseling while someone is still living, but grief counseling isn't just for post-life considerations; it can help you manage the intense sense of loss that can accompany a dementia diagnosis—not only the fear of losing the loved one as they were but also the ongoing grief as you witness your loved one's gradual decline. This type of counseling can be helpful when it comes to processing your feelings of loss and transitioning to new ways of relating to your loved one.

Family Therapy

Family therapy is another option that can improve communication and strengthen relationships among all family members. This form of therapy provides a safe space for each family member to express their fears, frustrations, and needs without judgment. In turn, this facilitates understanding by helping family members see each other's perspectives through a lens of empathy and cooperation. Through guided discussions and therapeutic exercises, your family can learn to manage the complexities of dementia together, supporting each other emotionally and practically.

Preparing for family therapy sessions, in particular, is key to maximizing their benefits. It can be helpful to come into each session with clear goals, such as improving communication, resolving conflicts, or simply gaining a better understanding of each family member's emotional experience. Being open to discussing difficult topics is also vital; therapy is a place to confront the hard truths and challenges that dementia brings. It can often be challenging to allow yourself to be vulnerable in front of others, which is why being prepared to be open and meet mutual goals is so helpful.

Finding the Right Therapist

You aren't going to mesh well with every therapist you find. Finding a therapist who you feel comfortable sharing your thoughts and feelings with is necessary, both for your comfort and for the sake of your mental health. As you look for the right therapist, it's important to seek out professionals who have experience with dementia patients and their families. Don't hesitate to ask a prospective therapist or counselor about their qualifications, their experience with dementia, and their approach to specific forms of therapy. You can find potential therapists through recommendations from your healthcare provider, local support groups, or online directories specializing in dementia care (Stanborough 2020).

THE ROLE OF SUPPORT GROUPS IN EMOTIONAL WELL-BEING

A support group and a support network are two different things. While a support *network* offers a web of people who you can rely on for support, a support *group* involves having a place to share and validate your emotions and those of other participants. Rather than being a group you call up or text for varying reasons (i.e., support, to hang out, to come over and help, and more), a support group is a place where people going through similar things can converge and aid each other in a neutral, pre-determined environment. Support groups, whether in-person or online, create an atmosphere where emotions and experiences can be shared and validated, which comes along with many benefits.

The benefits of a support group are multifaceted, including a sense of belonging, a reduction of feelings of isolation, and an outlet for expressing feelings that might be difficult to communicate with others who don't understand what you're going through. Furthermore, support groups can be a gold mine of practical advice, where you can find coping strategies and caregiving techniques that have been effective for others in similar situations. This first-hand experience and the knowledge stemming from it means that solutions are tried and tested, saving you time and stress.

Caregiving for a loved one with dementia is no easy task. The good news is that support groups vary widely in their focus and format, so it's possible to find one that meets your needs and preferences. Some groups are disease-specific, focusing solely on early-onset dementia, while others include various types of dementia or broader cognitive impairments. In-person meetings can provide a tangible sense of community and immediate personal connection. These groups typically meet in community centers, hospitals, or places of worship, providing a regular schedule that members can rely on. However, online forums and virtual meetings offer flexibility and accessibility, particularly beneficial for those who may have mobility challenges or live in areas with fewer in-person resources. These digital platforms can be greatly influential as well, as they ensure that support is just a click away, enabling participation from the comfort of your home at any time that suits your schedule (Friedman et al. 2018).

Starting a Support Group

If you find yourself in a place where support groups for early-onset dementia are lacking, starting your own group can be a rewarding act that fills this gap and creates a support system resource for others. Begin by reaching out to local health professionals, social workers, and community leaders to gauge interest and gather support—this can help you find professionals willing to offer support to the group. When it comes to finding a place to host the group, facilities like libraries, community centers, and places of worship often provide free or low-cost spaces for community support groups.

Of course, your support group has to have membership. Promoting your support group can be done through flyers, social media posts, and collaborations with local clinics or hospitals. As the group evolves, you can also work to obtain sponsorships from local businesses or health organizations that can help cover costs for materials and guest speakers, adding a professional edge to the group sessions.

With all of these aspects of maintaining emotional and psychological in mind, you have a clear roadmap for sustaining your mental health through coping strategies, seeking professional help, forming a support system, and more. Remember that no matter who you are, sustaining your mental health is the key to putting your best foot forward when it comes to managing dementia. Looking ahead, the next chapter will dig into practical caregiving strategies that can further enhance daily living and support for those navigating life with early-onset dementia, continuing our exploration of how to manage this condition with compassion and effectiveness.

5

PRACTICAL CAREGIVING STRATEGIES

As a caregiver, you face hurdles; it's an undeniable fact of the role. At the same time, it can be much simpler if you have practical caregiving strategies that empower you to support your loved one and help them feel safe. You might have concerns about how to keep their health and wellness consistent, how to manage behavioral challenges, and what you can do to offer your loved one comfort. This chapter dives into the significance of different practical strategies for caregiving that can help you achieve this, offering both respite and clarity to you and your loved ones.

ESTABLISHING EFFECTIVE ROUTINES FOR PATIENTS AND CAREGIVERS

Benefits of a Structured Routine

The creation of a structured daily routine is more than jotting down a schedule—it means creating a framework within which safety, familiarity, and predictability can be facilitated for your loved one. For people with early-onset dementia, routines provide a sense of familiarity in a world that becomes more and more unfamiliar with each passing day. The predictability of a routine can reduce stress and anxiety by a lot, which are often struggles people with dementia face as a result of not knowing what comes next. The routine doesn't just benefit your loved one, though; for caregivers, a routine alleviates the constant decision-making burden about daily activities and timings, making for a smoother, more manageable caregiving process.

Creating a Daily Schedule

When you create a daily schedule, you're anchoring daily activities to specific times. Routines based on a schedule can help align these activities with the times when your loved one feels most alert and engaged. For instance, if mornings are when your loved one feels the most energetic, then scheduling more demanding tasks like doctor's appointments, exercises, or social engagements during this time can make those interactions more successful and fulfilling. You should also take the time to understand which times of day tend to show energy dips or mood changes in your loved one, which can help you plan quieter, more restful activities appropriately.

Crafting a daily schedule tailored to your loved one's best times of day means that you can arrange tasks in a clear, convenient way. Once you know when your loved one is comfortable with high- and low-energy tasks, start creating that routine by mapping out the usual daily necessities—

meals, medication, and rest—and then build around these with activities that are both necessary and enjoyable. For example, regular meals should be incorporated at the same time each day to maintain nutritional health, and medication reminders should be set to align with these meals to create an easy-to-remember routine.

From there, include activities that your loved one finds meaningful and enjoyable in between those key activities. This could be anything from morning walks, which can help kickstart the day with energy, to afternoon crafts or reading sessions that allow for creativity and relaxation. The key is consistency; having these activities at the same time each day can enhance anticipation and participation. It is also beneficial to schedule regular check-ins or calls with friends and family, which gives your loved one something to look forward to ("Hobbies and Dementia Craftivism," n.d.).

Incorporating Flexibility

While the structure of a routine is helpful, the unpredictable nature of dementia means that some days may not go as planned. Adapting to these day-to-day variations in mood and ability means that you have to be flexible in order to offer the best care possible to your loved one. This might mean having a range of activities that can be swapped around depending on how the day is unfolding or allowing for longer periods of rest on days when fatigue sets in earlier. The goal is to balance structure with flexibility, creating a routine that respects your loved one's current state while still providing a framework that guides the day.

Routine as a Behavioral Management Tool

Outside of consistency, structured routines also serve as a powerful way to manage behavioral issues commonly associated with dementia, such as irritability or confusion. A predictable routine reduces anxiety by providing a familiar pattern of activities that orient your loved one to the time of day and expected behaviors. For example, an evening routine that includes dimming lights and soft music can signal that it is time to wind down, preparing them for bedtime and reducing sleep disturbances. Likewise, having set times for meals can reduce anxiety related to hunger or uncertainty about when food will be available ("Setting Routines and Reminders," n.d.).

NAVIGATING BEHAVIORAL CHANGES AND CHALLENGES

Continuing to think about the intricacies of caregiving for someone with early-onset dementia requires understanding and managing behavioral changes. The wide array of behavioral changes can be confusing and distressing, both for you and your loved one. While early-onset dementia is a bit different for each person, common behavioral shifts include increased aggression, wandering, and disturbances in sleep patterns.

Handling Aggression

Aggression is a common behavioral change that people with early-onset dementia face, and it can be troubling for caregivers if you aren't sure what to look for or how to manage it. Aggression may look like verbal outbursts or physical actions, and this often stems from frustration or confusion. Addressing the troubling behaviors of early-onset dementia —and as that dementia progresses—effectively means gaining a compassionate approach that focuses on understanding the root causes of such behaviors. From there, you can work toward implementing strategies to mitigate distress.

That said, there are a few things you can do to help manage your loved one's aggression. Creating a calm environment is crucial. This can be achieved by maintaining a quiet, uncluttered home that helps reduce anxiety and overstimulation— or by tailoring a specific room to be soothing in the face of aggression or distress. Soft lighting, comfortable furniture, and familiar objects can contribute to a sense of security and peace for your loved one. When aggressive behaviors occur, try to remain calm and avoid confrontation. Instead, acknowledge the emotion being expressed and try redirecting attention to a different, soothing activity like listening to favorite music or looking through a photo album. Remember that moments of aggression aren't personal; they arise from confusion, not from personal anger (Family Caregiver Alliance 2016).

Handling Wandering

Wandering is another troubling behavior that caregivers have to learn to manage. It can occur when your loved one feels restless or is searching for something but can't remember what that is. Redirecting their attention, just like with aggression, is also beneficial when it comes to the prevention of wandering. To facilitate this, engage your loved one in simple tasks that are fulfilling and within their capability, such as folding laundry or organizing a drawer. This can distract from the need to wander while helping them feel fulfilled *and* giving you some help with simple tasks. Ensuring that all basic needs are met—such as hunger, thirst, and the use of the restroom—can also prevent restlessness that leads to wandering. If wandering still persists or is a concern, safety measures like secure locks on doors and GPS tracking devices can be used to keep your loved one safe without being intrusive (Family Caregiver Alliance 2016).

Improving Sleep

It's common for people with dementia to experience sleep disturbances, such as insomnia or increased napping during the day. These disruptions can alter the body's natural circadian rhythms and exacerbate confusion, blurring the lines between day and night. You can help your loved one sleep better by helping them go to bed and wake up at the same time each day, which can regulate their understanding of day and night. It also helps to make their bedroom comfortable and organized and to leave a little bit of light on. This reduces anxiety and confusion. I also recommend keeping the bathroom light on so that they can easily find the bathroom without confusion, wandering, or getting injured (Family Caregiver Alliance 2016).

Communication for Behavioral Concerns

Effective communication plays a big role in managing behavioral changes. When conveying messages or instructions to your loved one, use simple choices and clear, short sentences to reduce the cognitive load they experience. This clarity helps minimize misunderstandings and frustrations. Maintaining a calm tone and a gentle pace in your speech is also important—it invites cooperation and reduces the likelihood of agitation. You can also use non-verbal cues, such as maintaining eye contact and reassuring touch, to convey empathy and understanding, which can be comforting during moments of confusion or distress (Family Caregiver Alliance 2016).

Considering Professional Advice

There might be instances where behavioral changes can be too challenging for you to manage on your own despite all your efforts. If this happens, seeking professional help from medical or behavioral specialists is a great idea. Specialists like geriatric psychiatrists, neurologists, or behavior therapists can provide assessments to understand the underlying causes of troubling behaviors and, from there, can recommend treatments to help. Treatments for behavioral problems can range from medication adjustments to specialized therapies.

ACTIVITIES OF DAILY LIVING: TIPS FOR FACILITATING INDEPENDENCE

For someone with early-onset dementia, independence can be a major challenge. At the same time, independence in daily activities is part of what your loved one needs to maintain quality of life. As a part of caregiving, it's important to help your loved one maintain as much independence as they can despite the progression of their disease.

Doing so begins with a careful and compassionate assessment of what activities of daily living (ADLs) your loved one can perform by themselves and which ones might require some assistance. ADLs include essential self-care tasks such as eating, dressing, grooming, and bathing. The objective here is not to highlight limitations but to identify opportunities where a bit of support could enable greater independence.

Assessing your loved one's abilities is a process of constant consideration. Thus, you should observe how your loved one manages tasks throughout the day and note any changes or difficulties. For example, your loved one might find dressing manageable but struggle with buttons or zippers. In eating, using standard cutlery might be challenging if coordination is an issue. Ongoing observation is crucial in tailoring support to your loved one's specific needs; it means that support needs can be observed and changed as your loved one changes.

It can make a big difference to your loved one if tools like zipper pulls, Velcro, and simple eating utensils are introduced, making everyday interactions easier. It's helpful if these modifications simplify the need for coordination, vision, and grip. Upon introducing assistive methods to your loved one's life, demonstrating how to use a dressing aid or the best way to utilize an adapted fork can empower them with the knowledge and confidence to use these tools effectively.

Outside of simplifying physical interactions, you can also help by breaking tasks into manageable steps. For instance, breaking down the task of getting dressed into a step-by-step process can make it less overwhelming and more manageable. Visual cues, such as labels or color-coded systems, can help remind your loved one of the steps involved in each task or where items are stored, which reduces frustration and enhances their ability to perform tasks independently. The most important part of fostering independence for your loved one is seeing where they struggle and accommodating that, all while encouraging engagement where they feel confident.

THE IMPORTANCE OF PERSONALIZED PATIENT-CENTERED CARE

The concept of patient-centered care is vital when it comes to addressing the medical symptoms of dementia. It goes above and beyond to honor and respond to the unique needs of the person experiencing these symptoms. This approach hinges on adapting care strategies to fit the personal preferences, needs, and values of each person rather than relying on a one-size-fits-all solution. The benefits of this tailored approach are a more humane and effective care plan, where the person with dementia is always at the heart of all decisions and actions.

One of the key elements of patient-centered care is the integration of the patient's life story into their care regime. In this case, you're aiming to bring your loved one's life story into their care plan in a meaningful way—their experiences don't simply fade with the onset of dementia. Understanding your loved one's background—such as their career, hobbies, likes, and dislikes—can enhance the caregiving experience. For instance, if your loved one was a former painter, they might find comfort and expression in having art supplies on hand, while a lifelong gardener might thrive on having access to a garden or plants to care for. Weaving these personal elements into daily care routines can invoke positive memories and emotions while fostering a sense of comfort that can be deeply reassuring for your loved one.

Monitoring and adjusting care is another important facet to consider in order to ensure that your loved one's care is effective and responsive to their evolving needs. Make sure to be mindful of how your loved one's behavior, health, and abilities are changing so that you can make modifications based on those considerations. For example, if your loved one once enjoyed group activities and now becomes overwhelmed by them due to the progression of their dementia, it might be appropriate to introduce more one-on-one interactions or quieter activities. Continually adapting the care plan to fit their needs means that you can continue to provide care that meets your loved one where they are, enhancing their quality of life at every stage of their condition ("The Role of Personalized Healthcare" 2024).

RESPITE CARE: UNDERSTANDING ITS IMPORTANCE AND HOW TO ACCESS IT

For a second, let's talk about you and your needs as a caregiver. You have a lot going on—caring for another human being is no small responsibility. It can lead to burnout, which we talked about earlier, and burnout means that you're not providing effective care because your brain is in a frenzy. Burnout exhausts your health, mentally and physically, and can make caregiving feel more like a burden than a loving responsibility. One of the most important ways that you can continue to care for your loved one while maximizing your own mental and physical health is through taking advantage of respite care.

Respite care is a vital service that can act as a lifeline for you as a caregiver. The point of respite care is to provide you with the necessary breaks to recharge and maintain your own health. It is, essentially, temporary relief that allows you to step away from your daily responsibilities for a few hours or days, all while remaining secure in the knowledge that your loved one is in safe hands.

There are several types of respite care services available, and each one is designed to accommodate different needs and situations:

- **In-Home Respite Care:** In-home respite care is a popular option, where a professional caregiver comes to your home to provide care. This means that you can leave the house for a while or simply take a break as someone else helps your loved one. This type of care can be especially comforting to the

person with dementia, as it allows them to stay in a familiar environment.
- **Adult Day Care Centers:** Adult day care centers offer another form of respite care. At the centers, social activities and care are provided in a professionally staffed group setting. This gives caregivers a break and provides valuable social interaction for the person with dementia.
- **Short-Term Residential Care:** For longer breaks, short-term residential care can allow your loved one to stay in a facility for a few days or weeks—where they receive 24-hour care—so that you have time for longer respite or vacations.
- **Coordinating with Caregivers:** While not a formal respite care arrangement, if you know other caregivers, respite care can be coordinated where one person monitors and assists both loved ones, and the responsibility is traded off.

While respite care can be convenient, it does require several practical steps to participate. For example, you should start by evaluating different respite care providers to find a reliable, honest facility or provider to trust with the care of your loved one. This can be done by visiting facilities, talking to staff, and checking references to make sure that each option you consider offers high-quality care for dementia patients. When considering in-home respite care instead of a facility, interviews with potential caregivers can help assess their compatibility and expertise. Furthermore, understanding the types of care each service offers, their operating hours, and the cost are important factors in choosing the right respite care option.

Funding for respite care is a common worry for many caregivers. Fortunately, there are many options you have that can help manage the costs. Long-term care insurance policies often cover some forms of respite care because respite care is a medical need, so reviewing your policy is a good first step. Medicaid may cover respite care for eligible individuals, and Veterans Affairs (VA) offers help for qualifying veterans. If these options aren't enough, many states have programs funded by the National Family Caregiver Support Program that can help provide respite care funding. Even local community organizations often have resources or grants that might make respite care more affordable to you.

In this chapter, we have thoroughly discussed the critical role of practical caregiving strategies in managing early-onset dementia, from establishing effective routines to understanding the incredible benefits of respite care. Each strategy that you've picked up is designed both to enhance the quality of life for your loved one with dementia and also to support you in your integral role in your loved one's day-to-day life. Shifting gears, it's time for us to dive deeper into what you can do to further support the quality of your loved one's life, even as their condition continues to decline. After all, they deserve the best—let's talk about how we can provide that.

6

ENHANCING QUALITY OF LIFE

As each day unfolds for your loved one, finding moments that spark joy and encourage engagement can transform their time living with early-onset dementia. It's common to think that people with dementia have a low-quality life, but by helping your loved one find therapeutic and health-centric activities that boost their physical abilities while revitalizing the mind, you can make sure that your loved one experiences days full of achievement and connection (Banerjee 2006). This chapter delves into the process of selecting enjoyable therapeutic and health-improving activities for your loved one that are beneficial in maintaining cognitive functions and personal skills.

THERAPEUTIC ACTIVITIES SUITABLE FOR EARLY-ONSET DEMENTIA

Selecting the right activities for someone with early-onset dementia means understanding the delicate balance between challenge and enjoyment. Activities that are fun but challenging give your loved one a sense of achievement, joy, and satisfaction that can offset the lull of each day's routine tasks. The key to balancing these considerations is to tailor these activities to match their cognitive level and interests. Activities that you choose should have the flexibility to adapt to changing abilities, allowing for modifications as needed without losing what makes them enjoyable. For instance, someone who enjoyed complex puzzles might now find simpler versions more manageable yet equally satisfying. There are many different types of activities to choose from, meaning that you and your loved one will certainly find something perfect for them.

Cognitive Stimulation Activities

Cognitive stimulation—keeping the brain active—is an important part of managing early-onset dementia because it helps your loved one maintain mental functions for as long as possible. Activities that challenge the mind, such as puzzles, games, and brain teasers, often involve problem-solving, memory, and processing skills that help maintain your loved one's daily cognitive functions. Simple crossword puzzles, matching games, or memory cards are just a few options that can provide just the right amount of challenge to stimulate your loved one without causing frustration. If you can help your loved one engage with these activities on a daily basis, it may just help slow the decline of their cognitive functions—all while offering them something fun to look forward to

Skill-Based Activities

Incorporating skill-based activities into your loved one's day can also be a source of great joy and self-esteem. Think about the skills that your loved one used to enjoy or excel at —finding an opportunity for these skills to make a comeback can awaken a sense of familiarity and competence that is truly uplifting. For example, if your loved one enjoyed cooking before their diagnosis, using simple recipes or asking them to help with simple kitchen tasks that are within their capabilities can be stimulating and positive. Gardening can be adapted by using container gardens or raised beds to reduce the physical strain while still providing the satisfaction of tending to plants. The bottom line is that any skill-based interest that your loved one had or has can be adapted through simplification, encouraging enjoyment at any stage.

Engagement Through Technology

Technology offers a unique opportunity for engagement for your loved one, bringing a world of possibilities into the comfort and safety of home. Tablets and computers can be used to play interactive games that are fun and support cognitive abilities. Apps designed specifically for dementia patients can include games that improve memory, problem-solving skills, and even hand-eye coordination. Games designed specifically for your loved one can meet them where they are and offer diverse activities that fit their individual preferences.

The Impact of Music and Art Therapy

It might sound unconventional, but music and art therapy have been shown to be incredibly effective as a tool for those experiencing early-onset dementia ("The Unexpected Benefits of Music Therapy for Dementia Patient," 2023). Music therapy, in particular, presents a ton of benefits, including emotional, cognitive, and social aspects. The power of music to evoke memories is unparalleled, tapping into long-seated recollections that might seem lost but can be vividly recalled with the right melody. Beyond that, engaging in music therapy can lead to significant moments of reconnection with past experiences and emotions, which leads to comfort and a sense of continuity. Moreover, the rhythmic and structured nature of music provides cognitive stimulation that can help maintain linguistic skills and improve mood.

If you think that music therapy might help your loved one, make it a part of their daily routine. In order to integrate music therapy into daily routines, try setting aside specific times for listening to music that your loved one enjoys or has emotional connections with. This could be a mix of soothing classical pieces, beloved old songs, or even new music that can prompt interest and engagement. Singing along or even moving to the music can further enhance the therapeutic effects by encouraging physical activity and expression.

Additionally, art therapy offers a complementary avenue for expression and cognitive engagement through visual and tactile mediums. It allows emotions and thoughts to be expressed in a non-verbal manner, which can be incredibly liberating for someone who struggles with language due to dementia. The act of creating something visually, whether it's painting, drawing, or sculpting, can provide a sense of accomplishment and pride. For people with dementia, art therapy sessions can include simple coloring books, finger painting, or clay modeling, which are not only manageable but also deeply satisfying. These activities stimulate fine motor skills and cognitive functions like planning and decision-making, contributing to a richer daily experience ("6 Ways That Art Therapy Can Help People with Memory Loss | Lesley University," n.d.).

Documenting Therapy Progress

As your loved one engages with different therapeutic exercises and tasks, monitoring and documenting their process should always be considered. When you or their therapist do so, it's easier to tailor future sessions to their likes and dislikes. Also, observing progress or preference changes can be instrumental in monitoring the progression of dementia as a whole.

To track their progress, it's helpful to keep a simple log or journal where you note the types of music or art activities that evoke the most positive responses in your loved one. You can even encourage them to talk to you about their experiences to ensure that you fully understand your observations. And speaking of, the observations you make can include emotional reactions, levels of engagement, or any spontaneous memories or conversations that arise during the sessions. This documentation helps you understand what works best and what might need adjustment so that each future session is as fulfilling and beneficial as possible.

Interactive Element: Reflective Journaling Prompt

Consider this an invitation to reflect on the activities that currently fill your loved one's days. Which of these activities brings them the most joy and a sense of accomplishment? Have you asked which ones they enjoy? Are there past hobbies or interests that could be reintroduced into their routine, perhaps in a modified form? Taking a moment to write down these reflections can help you identify the types of activities that your loved one might find the most meaningful and enjoyable.

SOCIAL ENGAGEMENT: KEEPING CONNECTED WITH THE COMMUNITY

Maintaining relationships with friends and family, despite the progression of dementia, is non-negotiable when it comes to fostering emotional health and a sense of belonging. Regular interactions can help combat feelings of isolation and provide continuous emotional support, which is invaluable in the face of dementia. However, while social engagement is a fundamental aspect of well-being for anyone with dementia, it's not always easy for your loved one to facilitate these connections on their own. Helping your loved one keep in touch is a rewarding way for them to stay connected as you improve their quality of life.

Scheduling Social Engagements

One effective strategy to help your loved one sustain social relationships is regular scheduling. Setting specific times for phone calls, video chats, or visits can create a routine that helps your loved one stay connected. These scheduled interactions become something that they can look forward to, which improves their overall comfort and consistency. Try scheduling these visits for high-energy times of day, when your loved one can get the most out of each interaction—and so that they can show up as the best version of themselves to each interaction. If these events are outside of the home, try to arrange to leave early or have extra time to get ready so that your loved one doesn't feel stressed or rushed.

Using Technology

The advent of technology, particularly social media and video calls, has transformed the way we maintain relationships—making it easier for your loved one to stay in touch even from a distance. Platforms like Facebook, Skype, or Zoom can allow your loved one to participate in real-time conversations and share moments with others regardless of physical location. These tools are especially helpful if your loved one struggles with leaving the home or engaging with others but still wishes to communicate. Helping set up these tools and making them easy for your loved one to see and use (i.e., increasing the font size or setting it up so that their contacts are always visible) can also make independent social interactions simpler.

Community Engagement

Just like personal interactions are importance, community engagement is equally vital. When people with dementia engage with their community, it means that they have the chance to connect with a broader circle and enjoy social activities revolving around their interests and needs. Many communities now offer programs and activities specifically designed to be inclusive for individuals with cognitive challenges. For example, special movie screenings with adjusted sound levels and lighting, museum tours that are slower paced with more seating, or local community events with designated quiet areas can make social outings more enjoyable and less stressful for people going through challenges like dementia. Making it so that your loved one can participate in these activities can improve their social life and the quality of their life overall.

Volunteering

For some people with dementia, it can be hard to get out and about or do non-essential activities like volunteering; however, for people who still have a full range of motion and the cognitive ability to do so, engaging in volunteer work can equate to a sense of purpose and connection with the community. Many organizations value the contributions of individuals with diverse experiences, including those with dementia, so your loved one will almost always be welcomed. Simple volunteer activities, such as assisting at a local food bank, participating in community clean-ups, or engaging in peer support roles, can be adapted to match your loved one's current abilities. These activities mean that your loved one can give back, build new relationships, and maintain a sense of self-worth and accomplishment.

Advocating on Their Behalf

It's not always the case that your loved one can advocate for themselves when activities or places aren't accessible for them. Creating or advocating for a dementia-friendly community is a powerful way you can strive to enhance the inclusivity and accessibility of your local environment, helping not just your loved one but others like them. This might look like contributing to initiatives such as training local businesses and public service providers on how to interact effectively with people with dementia or improve physical accessibility in public areas. By participating in or supporting these initiatives, you help create a community that understands dementia and honors the needs of those with dementia.

PHYSICAL EXERCISE AND ITS BENEFITS TO COGNITIVE HEALTH

Enhancing your loved one's quality of life means also embracing physical exercise as a part of their daily routine. As a caregiver, it's up to you to help your loved one remain active, which is no insignificant task—remaining physically active for as long as possible can improve their cognitive and physical well-being.

Types of Activity

Not all forms of physical activity are built equal, but luckily, there are many types of activity that are perfect for those with dementia. Your loved one is bound to find a form of exercise that is accommodating and enjoyable. You have a few options for where you can begin when it comes to exploring opportunities for your loved one to exercise:

- **Walking:** Walking is one of the most accessible forms of exercise. Perhaps the best part about walking is its flexibility. The pace and duration of walks can be streamlined to fit your loved one's comfort level. Whether it's a gentle stroll through your neighborhood or a more structured walk in a local park, walking supports cardiovascular health, which is crucial for maintaining blood flow to the brain and, therefore, cognitive functions ("8 Ways Walking Can Boost Your Brain Health," n.d.). You can't go wrong with walking!
- **Swimming:** Swimming is another excellent low-impact exercise, perfect for those who might find joint strain or coordination an issue with other types of workouts. The buoyancy of water reduces stress on the body, allowing for a comprehensive workout that feels more like relaxation rather than exertion ("5 Benefits of Swimming for Seniors Who Need Alzheimer's Care | Richmond West," n.d.).
- **Tai Chi:** Tai chi, often referred to as meditation in motion, synthesizes slow, deliberate movements with deep breathing, thus enhancing physical balance and mental focus ("A Sharper Mind: Tai Chi Can Improve Cognitive Function" 2020).
- **Group Exercise Classes:** For a more social exercise experience, group exercise classes designed for seniors or individuals with cognitive challenges can be both uplifting and supportive. They also serve as an opportunity to maintain social connections and

experience physical activity in a structured setting (Long et al. 2020).

Making it Routine

Incorporating exercise, no matter which form, into your loved one's daily routine should be a deliberate choice. Aiming to align physical activity with your loved one's best times of day and any existing schedules you both have. This mindful integration makes exercise a natural part of their day rather than a burden. Outside of picking exercises that are easy, make sure to offer activities that cater to your loved one's interests—such as choosing nature walks if they enjoy the outdoors or water aerobics if they love being in the pool. This can increase their motivation and ability to enjoy exercise, making it more likely that they'll cooperate and find fulfillment from it. If possible, it's also beneficial to vary their activities to keep the routine engaging and cover different aspects of physical health, from endurance and flexibility to balance and strength.

Health Benefits

If you're wondering why I'm so adamant about exercise, it's because regular physical activity is incredibly beneficial for cognitive health. As mentioned earlier, exercise enhances blood flow throughout the body, including the brain, which is essential for maintaining and forming new neural connections. Improved blood flow can lead to better brain function, helping to slow the progression of cognitive decline associated with dementia. Exercise also plays a crucial role in mood regulation; it stimulates the release of endorphins, often known as the body's natural mood elevators (Better Health Channel 2021). This release can help combat feelings of depression and anxiety, which are common in people dealing with dementia. Furthermore, maintaining an exercise routine can contribute to better sleep patterns, which in itself is a critical factor in cognitive health. Good quality sleep helps consolidate memories and clear the brain of toxins, supporting overall cognitive functions. All of these benefits are perfect for someone with early-onset dementia.

Safety Considerations

Safety is always important to think about when planning an exercise routine, especially for people with dementia. Always consider that your loved one will need proper supervision during physical activities in order to keep them safe and supported. It's important to avoid overexertion; activities should be challenging enough to provide a benefit but not so strenuous as to cause discomfort or fatigue. Have your loved one start slowly, especially if they are new to regular exercise, and gradually increase the intensity and duration of their workouts as their fitness improves—or reduce to accommodate dementia-related changes. Special attention should be given to preventing falls during exercise, which can be common for people with declining mobility. Choosing safe environments, using appropriate equipment, and perhaps modifying exercises to reduce the risk of balance-related incidents are all great considerations for keeping your loved one safe. For instance, tai chi can be adapted to be performed while seated, still offering the benefits of the exercise but minimizing the risk of falling.

PLANNING FOR MEANINGFUL OUTINGS AND VISITS

Exploring the world outside the confines of home means that your loved one has a chance to refresh their scenery and gain experiences that can be especially beneficial for them. Many people with dementia stay inside for the duration of their disease, which isn't necessary if they can get out and about.

Picking a Location

Not all outings are going to be suitable for your loved one. Choosing destinations that are both secure and stimulating should be your biggest consideration when planning outings that improve your loved one's quality of life. Nature parks are a great choice; they provide a serene environment where you and your loved one can enjoy the calming effects of green spaces and gentle walks. Art galleries are another fantastic choice, giving your loved one a visually stimulating experience that can spark memories and inspire conversations about the displayed artworks. Additionally, community events that include sensory-friendly environments can be enjoyed by your loved one as they are often designed to accommodate individuals with sensory processing sensitivities, something your loved one might be prone to.

Pre-Outing Preparations

Unlike earlier years, going on an outing when you have dementia isn't as simple as walking out the door—your loved one needs some help from you. Preparing for an outing involves several considerations to make sure that everything is smooth and enjoyable. Transportation needs to be planned first; it's important to arrange for safe and comfortable means of travel for your loved one. If you're driving, for example, the vehicle should be comfortable, and the drive time is within the tolerable limit for your loved one. If public transportation is needed, it should be used during off-peak hours to avoid your loved one feeling overwhelmed or confused.

Packing necessary items is also essential; these might include medications, sun hats, comfortable shoes, water bottles, and any necessary emergency contact information. A checklist can be helpful to ensure nothing is forgotten in the rush to head out. Try to let your loved one carry items that can be replaced if lost—like their own water bottle, if possible—to promote independence on outings.

Incorporating Familiarity and Variety

Balancing familiarity with new experiences is key to a successful outing. Visiting familiar places can be comforting and reduce anxiety, elevating your loved one's enjoyment of the outing. However, introducing new experiences is equally important because it can stimulate the mind and provide fresh topics for thought and engagement. This might include visiting a new exhibit at a familiar museum or trying a different path in a well-loved park. The key is to introduce new experiences gradually and gauge their response to see if they are finding joy in the experience instead of feeling overwhelmed.

Reflecting on Outings

Reflecting on the outings you take your loved one on after the fact can help you gain valuable insights into what worked well and what might need adjustment for future excursions. This reflection should involve direct feedback from your loved one, if possible, as their input can help you understand their experience. Did they enjoy the activity? Were they comfortable during transportation? Were there aspects of the outing that caused discomfort?

As we close this chapter on enhancing the quality of life for your loved one, remember that each outing, each activity, and each new experience plays a vital role in enriching their life as someone with early-onset dementia. The thoughtful planning and execution of these enhancements only serves to highlight your commitment to providing a life full of enriching experiences that lead to joy, engagement, and continued growth.

As we transition from discussing daily activities and outings to the broader aspects of dementia care, the next chapter will delve into advanced care planning—such as evolving care to meet the evolving needs of your loved one as early-onset dementia progresses.

7

ADVANCED CARE PLANNING

Wading through the ebbs and flows of early-onset dementia is more than simply adapting to daily changes; it also includes preparing for the future stages of this condition. Understanding what lies ahead can be lifesaving during times of uncertainty, granting you clarity and direction as you adjust your care strategies to meet the ever-changing needs of your loved one. This chapter focuses on the later stages of dementia, a period that may seem daunting but, with the right preparation, can be approached with knowledge, empathy, and compassion.

UNDERSTANDING AND PREPARING FOR THE LATER STAGES OF DEMENTIA

As dementia progresses, the later stages can present challenges that are significantly different from the early or middle stages. Typically characterized by increased memory loss, severe disorientation, and substantial changes in physical capabilities, these later stages require a deeper level of care and understanding since your loved one loses a significant amount of independence. In addition, memory loss becomes more pronounced, with individuals possibly unable to recall significant life events or even recognize close family members. Disorientation also increases, which can lead to difficulties in understanding time and place, potentially resulting in distress and anxiety. Physical abilities decline as well, and challenges in mobility and the performance of daily activities become more prevalent.

It's necessary that you recognize these changes as part of the disease's progression and not as the personal failings of your loved one. Each symptom reflects significant changes occurring in their brain, all of which impact memory, thinking, and physical abilities. Understanding these symptoms can help you anticipate the needs that arise and adjust how you care for your loved one accordingly. For example, increased memory loss may necessitate the use of more visual aids around the home or more frequent reminders of daily routines and personal history (Alzheimer's Society 2019).

Care Needs Assessment

Assessing the care needs of your loved one is one way to really understand how you can best support your loved ones. Assessing the care needs during these stages requires considering around-the-clock supervision to ensure safety and meet the increasing demands of daily living. It's important to get a good idea of what and when your loved one struggles, enabling you to make decisions for their care that leave nothing to chance.

This assessment could lead to realizing the need for professional caregiving support or considering a residential care facility that can provide 24-hour care. Daily activities such as eating, dressing, and personal hygiene will likely require assistance at some point, and ensuring a safe environment becomes paramount to prevent accidents or injuries. It can be hard to do this on your own 24/7, so don't be afraid to consider full-time care facilities or hospice when the time comes.

Communication with Healthcare Providers

During the later stages of dementia, it's essential to maintain regular communication with your loved one's healthcare providers. Discussing your loved one's care plan in an ongoing manner facilitates quick and effective adjustments in response to the progression of the disease and any new health issues that arise. Moreover, healthcare providers can offer valuable insights and recommendations that help you manage their symptoms more effectively and improve comfort during their time spent with you. They can help guide decisions about changes in medication, the introduction of therapies, and the coordination of care among different health professionals as well, making them indispensable.

Emotional Preparation

For families and caregivers, preparing emotionally for the later stages of dementia is as important as preparing practically. Witnessing the decline in a loved one's cognitive abilities and physical health can be heartbreaking and devastating. Emotional preparation for this decline means acknowledging the difficulties of it and seeking support when needed. Support groups, counseling, and family therapy can be helpful as you work through the later stages of your loved one's dementia and the feelings that encompass it.

WHEN TO CONSIDER MEMORY CARE FACILITIES

Deciding to transition a loved one to a memory care facility can be one of the most challenging decisions you face during the course of caring for your loved one. It signifies the end of your journey as a caregiver, and that alone can be hard to accept. But beyond that, transitioning your loved one to such a facility means that you no longer have a constant watch over them, which can induce anxiety. It's a hard consideration to make, but one that's worthwhile at a certain point.

Understanding what a memory care facility is can help ease some of your stress about making the decision. Memory care facilities are specifically designed to cater to the needs of people with various forms of dementia. They maintain a structured environment that significantly minimizes stress and confusion for residents. One of the primary benefits of such facilities is their targeted programs that enhance the daily lives of patients. Such programs often include activities meant to stimulate memory, improve cognitive function, and maintain physical health, all within a safe and secure environment that prevents wandering and other common risks associated with dementia.

Memory care facilities aren't nursing homes; they offer specialized care that goes beyond what traditional nursing homes provide. The staff in memory care facilities are trained specifically to provide dementia-related care, which means that they understand the unique challenges and needs of those living with the condition. As a result, all aspects of care—from administering medications correctly to offering appropriate cognitive therapies—are handled by knowledgeable professionals who understand how to communicate effectively and compassionately with dementia patients. The environment in these facilities is also meticulously designed to reduce agitation and enhance comfort, incorporating features like secure walking paths, visual aids, and private spaces that allow for personalization, making residents feel more at home ("What Is Memory Care?" 2023).

Because memory care facilities can often be incredibly pricey, and not all accept Medicaid or insurance, you should also consider nursing facilities or nursing homes that do accept the insurance that your loved one has. These facilities also offer around the clock care and can be easier to afford if a memory care facility isn't a good fit for your loved one.

Evaluating Facilities

When considering a memory care or other facility, you need to conduct thorough evaluations of a few different facilities to find one that you feel will meet your loved one's needs. Begin by looking into the qualifications of the staff and the ratios of staff to residents. A higher number of well-trained staff members per resident typically equates to a higher level of personalized care. Safety features are also good to look for; check for secure exits and entrances, well-lit environments, and non-slip floors. Additionally, see if you can gather feedback from current residents and their families regarding their experiences—either by asking around or by checking online reviews for the facility.

In addition, I highly recommend that you visit the facilities you're considering personally to give you a better perspective on how they operate. During these visits, pay close attention to the interactions between staff and residents. Is the staff patient and respectful, and do the residents seem content and engaged? Also, review the daily activity schedule. Is there a concrete, simple, yet effective schedule? Are the activities suitable and beneficial for someone with dementia? Do they vary regularly to keep residents stimulated and active? This information can help you see what the day-to-day operations and the quality of care provided in that facility are like resulting in more informed decisions ("What to Look for When Searching for a Memory Care Facility" 2021).

Timing for Transition

So, when should you actually move your loved one to a memory care facility? Determining the right time to move a loved one can be based on several factors. If you think it might be time, ask yourself a few questions:

- Is it still safe for your loved one to be at home?
- Are their care needs beyond what family and home caregivers can provide?
- Are you able to continue providing the necessary level of care without compromising your health?

- Could a care facility improve your loved one's quality of life beyond what you can offer right now, either via social interactions, routine, or care?

If safety becomes an issue, or if the physical and emotional demands of caregiving are too great, it may be time to consider a transition. Furthermore, if your loved one's medical needs are complex and require professional health monitoring, a memory care facility can provide the necessary medical support.

Visitation and Ongoing Involvement

Maintaining an active role in your loved one's care after the transition is absolutely something that you can—and should—do. Regular visits can help ease the adjustment for both you and your loved one. These visits can be a comforting reminder of familiarity and love, which can be positive in influence as your loved one adjusts to the new environment. Also, actively participating in care planning meetings can ensure that your loved one's needs are being met and that their care plan continues to align with their health and personal preferences.

PALLIATIVE CARE OPTIONS AND DISCUSSIONS

You do have options for care outside of memory care facilities. Palliative care focuses on providing relief from the symptoms and stress of the disease by emphasizing comfort and quality of life rather than cure. This type of care is comprehensive, both addressing physical symptoms and attending to emotional, social, and spiritual needs. Because of its scope and focus, palliative care can help maintain the dignity and comfort of your loved one as they navigate the complexities of their condition ("Palliative Care and Dementia," n.d.).

Before we talk about how you can integrate palliative care into your loved one's treatment, addressing common misconceptions about palliative care is a must. It is often thought that palliative care is only for those who are in the final stages of life. However, this is not the case. Palliative care can be beneficial at various stages of an illness, including early stages, where it can serve to manage symptoms and maintain comfort as the disease progresses. It's important to understand that opting for palliative care does not mean giving up hope but rather choosing to focus on the quality of life and comfort for your loved one.

Discussing Palliative Care

Opening up conversations about palliative care can be sensitive. When considering this for your loved one with dementia, approach the discussion with clarity and compassion. Start by gathering all necessary information about the options and benefits of palliative care so that you're prepared for the conversation. Then, during the conversation, strive to maintain an atmosphere that is straightforward and respectful, keeping in mind their ability to understand and process the information—they might appreciate simple or complex discussions based on where their progression of dementia is at. As you discuss palliative care oprtions with your loved one, focus on how palliative care aims to improve quality of life and provide comfort, rather than on the progression of the disease, to put a positive spin on this treatment option. This will make it easier for your loved one to digest and agree to. If you're discussing this option with family members who might be hesitant, make it a point to discuss the goals of palliative care to alleviate fears and anxiety that they may have.

Integrating Palliative Care

Integrating palliative care into your loved one's existing care plan should be a carefully coordinated process. Doing so requires the collaboration of all healthcare providers helping your loved one so that everyone is on the same page regarding the goals and methods of care. This might include regular meetings with doctors, nurses, and specialists who are part of the care team as well, ensuring that you and each professional understand every aspect of your loved one's needs.

END-OF-LIFE CARE: MAKING DECISIONS WITH DIGNITY

Approaching end–of–life care from the starting point of early-onset dementia requires careful consideration. It is a shift that calls for compassion, understanding, and respect for the wishes of your loved one. Advance directives and living wills play a pivotal role in this phase, serving as a voice for individuals when they might no longer articulate their desires about their care. These documents are crucial in ensuring that the medical treatments provided align with the personal values and preferences of your loved one, thereby safeguarding their dignity at a vulnerable time.

Advance directives and living wills are legal tools that outline a person's wishes regarding medical treatments and interventions at the end of life, which we discussed in Chapter 2. They come into play when an individual can no longer communicate their decisions due to medical conditions, ensuring that their preferences for healthcare are known and respected. For example, some may choose to decline certain life-prolonging treatments if the quality of life would be severely compromised, while others might opt for all possible measures to extend life, regardless of the condition.

Comfort Measures

When curative treatment—an approach that helps alleviate or slow symptomatic progression—is no longer an option, the focus of care often shifts to comfort measures, which are interventions aimed at alleviating symptoms and ensuring that your loved one remains as comfortable as possible during the final stages of dementia. Pain management, for example, is a common component of these measures—it can effectively address the physical discomfort many dementia patients experience, like pain, confusion, and more.

Beyond managing pain, end-of-life care also focuses on creating a peaceful environment. You can help do this by personalizing the room of your loved one with items that bring comfort, such as family photos, favorite blankets, or a soothing playlist of cherished songs. Maintaining a quiet atmosphere, where disturbances are minimized, helps maintain a calm setting. Simple acts like keeping the lighting soft, managing room temperature, and checking to see that your loved one is in a comfortable position can significantly enhance their comfort during the end of their care ("How to Provide Additional Comfort at End of Life" 2022).

Ethical Considerations

End-of-life decision-making also involves a spectrum of ethical considerations that can be challenging if you're not sure of what to consider. For example, many families and caregivers struggle to find a balance between prolonging life and maintaining quality of life. Keeping your loved one alive doesn't always mean that that life is dignifying, which is why assessing whether continued treatment aligns with the patient's wishes is vital. You also have to think about issues around autonomy and your loved one's right to participate in decisions about their care, even as their cognitive abilities decline. In these situations, previously expressed wishes, documented in advance through methods we discussed in Chapter 2, can guide you.

THE ROLE OF HOSPICE IN MANAGING ADVANCED DEMENTIA

Finally, there's the matter of hospice to consider. Hospice care, distinct in its approach, centers on providing palliative treatment, which focuses on the comfort and quality of life for patients, specifically in the final stages of their illness. Unlike other medical care, the goal is not to cure but to offer peace and dignity, managing symptoms so that the individual's remaining time can be as comfortable and meaningful as possible.

Qualifying for Hospice

Typically, eligibility for hospice is determined by a physician's prognosis, generally indicated when a patient is expected to live six months or less if the disease follows its usual course ("Eligibility Guidelines" n.d.). The progression of dementia often meets this criterion, so when your loved one is close to the end of their life, they will likely qualify. The process to qualify and get into a hospice program usually involves assessments by healthcare providers specializing in hospice care, who will evaluate your loved one's overall health and ability to benefit from this type of palliative approach. With that said, obtaining hospice services will start with a referral from your loved one's primary care physician or neurologist, who can initiate those necessary evaluations and documentation we just talked about. From there, a hospice care center can support you through its unique process.

Services Provided by Hospice

Hospice care is renowned for its comprehensive range of services, and understanding those services can help alleviate some of the anxiety you may be feeling at the time of transitioning your loved one to such care. Hospice care is designed to address the varied needs of patients and their families, as well as provide round-the-clock medical care for your loved one—thanks to the services of a team of healthcare professionals skilled in end-of-life care. This team often includes doctors, nurses, and hospice aides, all coordinated to ensure that medical needs are met compassionately and efficiently.

Emotional support is another aspect of hospice care, provided through counseling services available to both patients and their families. This support helps in navigating the multifaceted emotions that arise during this time through guidance and understanding. Spiritual counseling is also available if desired, addressing the existential questions and needs that may emerge based on your family's beliefs and preferences (BAYADA Home Health Care 2019).

Navigating the Transition to Hospice

Transitioning to hospice care is an impactful step for families and can be filled with emotional distress if not handled carefully. Preparing for this transition involves both logistical and emotional preparation. Logistically, you should work closely with hospice providers to understand the scope of services offered by the facility and how they will be integrated into your loved one's existing care plan. This might involve home modifications to accommodate medical equipment or schedules to coordinate in-home care visits if hospice care is taking place inside the home. If not, discussions might center around when the transition will take place and what, in particular, your loved one needs.

Emotionally, preparing for hospice can be difficult. Open discussions with family members about the goals and expectations of hospice care can alleviate some anxieties and misunderstandings about hospice in general. It's also wise to engage in counseling services offered by hospice organizations, which can help families process their feelings about the transition and the impending loss of their loved one.

The later stages of managing dementia for your loved one can be some of the hardest to bear. It comes along with transitions in your daily life that are undeniable—often ones that signal the devastating end of your loved one's life. It's no easy consideration, but knowing what to expect and how you can ensure that your loved one is cared for does much to ease the emotional stress you're feeling.

Now, let's shift gears for a moment. People with dementia are often misunderstood or misrepresented, and socially, it's hard for people to understand and accommodate dementia-related needs due to stigma surrounding the disease ("Stigma against Dementia," n.d.). Becoming an advocate and involving yourself in the community—whether you're a caregiver, family member, or person with dementia yourself—can make a world of difference for those struggling with the condition.

8

ADVOCACY AND COMMUNITY INVOLVEMENT

Imagine a world where people don't have to worry about whether their loved one will be judged for having dementia, or whether the right care will be offered. In this world, accommodation is a certainty, shifting how those with dementia are treated and perceived. This is the future that advocacy can create, not just for those with dementia but for all people experiencing age, cognitive, or ability-related changes. Advocacy isn't just about speaking up; it deals with creating waves of change that ripple through communities, influence policies, and bring forth a deeper understanding and better support systems for individuals and families navigating this challenging path. Now, it's time to take a look at how you—yes, you—can become an advocate.

BECOMING A DEMENTIA ADVOCATE: STEPS AND STRATEGIES

Understanding Advocacy

Advocacy in the context of dementia carries out several pivotal roles. It involves raising awareness, not just to inform but to engender empathy and support from the broader community. Advocacy also influences policy to make sure that the needs and rights of those with dementia are considered in healthcare planning and community services. Advocacy even supports individuals and families directly by granting them a voice and a platform to share their experiences and challenges, thus contributing to a more informed and compassionate society.

The role of an advocate often begins with a personal connection to dementia, driven by the desire to make a difference in the lives of those affected. Whether you are someone with dementia, a caregiver, or simply a concerned community member, your voice can help illuminate the realities of living with dementia and guide efforts to improve care, support, and understanding.

Building a Platform

Establishing a credible advocacy platform is one of the first steps in establishing effective advocacy. This process means that you should identify the key messages that you want to convey that are relevant to your platform. For example, you can ask yourself what aspects of dementia need more awareness in your opinion—such as the early signs, the daily challenges, or perhaps the policy gaps in healthcare services.

Your target audience is equally important in building a platform for your advocacy efforts. Are you reaching out to policymakers, the general public, or other families dealing with dementia? Each audience requires a different approach in terms of language, channels, and content to truly speak to that group. For instance, policymakers may need detailed reports and data to listen and understand your point, while the general public might respond better to personal stories and simple facts that they can relate to.

Beyond that, effective communication strategies are the backbone of your advocacy efforts and platform. This includes everything from public speaking and writing articles to engaging in community discussions and online forums. Each method has its strengths and can reach different segments of your audience. Combining various strategies often yields the best results and allows you to spread your message widely and effectively.

Engaging with Local Organizations

Connecting with local dementia organizations can amplify your advocacy efforts. These organizations often have established platforms and networks that can help disseminate your message more widely. Collaboration can also lead to shared resources, whether it's access to the latest research, platforms for speaking publicly, or support in organizing community events.

To engage effectively, start by identifying the organizations in your area that focus on dementia. Reach out to them to explore potential collaborations. This could be anything from co-hosting awareness events to participating in advocacy campaigns. Such partnerships extend your reach and strengthen the collective impact of advocacy efforts, making a more substantial difference in the community.

Personal Storytelling

One of the most powerful tools in your advocacy toolkit is personal storytelling. Sharing your own experiences or those of your loved ones can make the abstract realities of dementia more palpable for others. Stories resonate in a way that statistics and general information do not; they touch hearts and inspire action.

To share your stories effectively and respectfully, consider the privacy and dignity of everyone involved. Obtain consent if you're sharing someone else's story, and be honest but considerate, avoiding overly graphic details that might distress or offend your listeners. Instead, focus on conveying the emotions and lessons learned from the experiences.

When sharing your story, focus on the emotional journey as well as the practical aspects of living with dementia. Describe the challenges but also highlight moments of joy and triumph. This balanced narrative helps in painting a full picture of what it's like to live with dementia, fostering a deeper understanding and stronger empathy among your audience.

USING SOCIAL MEDIA TO CONNECT AND EDUCATE OTHERS

In such a digitally driven era, social media platforms like Facebook, Twitter (X), and Instagram have become incredible tools for advocacy and education, especially in the context of early-onset dementia. These platforms lead to unique opportunities to spread awareness and connect with others who are navigating similar challenges. For instance, Facebook contributes a space for creating community groups where people can share their individual experiences and support each other, while Twitter's fast-paced environment is excellent for quick updates and links to more comprehensive resources. Simultaneously, Instagram, with its visual focus, can be used to share moving images and stories that capture the human side of living with dementia.

Content Creation

If you want to create content that engages and informs people about the highs and lows of dementia, you have to find a balance between authenticity and strategy. Start by considering the visuals—these are often the first elements that catch the eye. Photos and graphics that depict real-life scenarios, infographics that simplify complex information about dementia, or short videos that share personal stories can be highly effective.

Utilizing hashtags is another strategic tool that can increase the visibility of your posts. Hashtags like #DementiaAwareness, #KnowDementia, or #EarlyOnsetDementia can help your content reach a broader audience who are searching for related information, while tags like #MentalHealthAwareness can shed light on aspects of health that people often neglect to acknowledge. Additionally, sharing personal narratives or anecdotes online can make your posts more relatable and memorable. These stories turn dementia from a medical diagnosis to something people realize is very real and very human, which encourages a deeper connection with your audience ("Virtually Support World Alzheimer's Month," n.d.).

Building Community

Building an online community around dementia advocacy requires consistent engagement, so be sure that this is a commitment that you can follow through on. Regular posting keeps the community active and informed, while responding to comments and messages can help build trust and rapport with your followers. It's also helpful to collaborate with other advocacy accounts or influencers in the dementia space. These collaborations can include joint campaigns, shared posts, or even online events, all of which can amplify your message and extend your reach.

Considering Reach and Effectiveness

Of course, advocacy is meant to be effective. Whether your goal is to spread awareness, change social attitudes, or anything else, knowing how effective your efforts are can help you change your approach, keep up with new trends for spreading awareness, and more.

In order to gauge the reach and efficacy of your social media efforts, it's important to utilize the analytics tools provided by these platforms. Most social media sites offer basic analytics that track the reach and engagement of your posts, such as the number of likes, shares, comments, and views. Monitoring these metrics allows you to see which types of content resonate most with your audience, helping you refine your strategy and focus more on what works. For instance, if you notice that posts with personal stories generate more engagement, you might decide to feature more such stories in your future content.

ORGANIZING COMMUNITY EVENTS AND FUNDRAISERS

Another form of advocacy and community participation that you can work with is organizing community events and fundraisers. This can be a moving, positive way to raise both awareness and funds for early-onset dementia, all while making a difference in the lives of people with the condition. The successful planning and execution of events like these rely on careful organization and a deep understanding of the cause you are championing. Let's explore the foundational steps involved in bringing a community event or fundraiser to life, from the initial concept to the final execution.

Planning Community Events or Fundraisers

The journey of event planning begins with concept development, where you define the main purpose of the event—are you aiming to raise awareness, funds, or both? Once your purpose is clear, brainstorming ideas that align with your goals is a great next step. For example, if the aim is to educate the public about early-onset dementia, an educational seminar or workshop could be effective. On the other hand, if fundraising is the primary goal, a charity walk or gala dinner might be more appropriate to reach your goal. Each type of event has unique pros, cons, and logistical requirements, so choosing an event that matches your intention and ability to see it through is imperative.

Next, venue selection has to be considered when it comes to the practical planning of the event. The choice of venue should reflect the event's tone and purpose while also comfortably accommodating your expected number of attendees. Accessibility is key, especially considering the needs of those who might be living with early-onset dementia or other disabilities who may attend. Even if they don't attend, finding an accessible venue sends a strong message of inclusion no matter the time or place. Venues that are comfortable, spacious, and quiet are best for conversational meetings, while more energetic venues should be reserved for events that require that high energy.

Naturally, budgeting for your event can't be overlooked, even if you're fundraising. Creating a detailed budget early on helps in managing expenses and ensures that the event remains financially viable. This budget should include estimates for venue rental, catering, security, insurance, and any other logistical needs. If the budget exceeds the amount of income expected from donations or the amount you can allocate to the event, then it's worthwhile to consider changes that make your event more feasible.

Finally, let's talk logistics. Logistics form the framework that supports the entire event. This includes everything from the flow of the event (i.e., which topics will be covered in which order during a workshop), timing, registration processes, and the setup of any necessary equipment. Ensuring that all these elements work together cohesively makes for a smoother, more impactful event. You can make sure that your event is clear and logical by running through the entire event schedule beforehand to anticipate any potential issues and plan contingencies for any mishaps you may encounter (OneCause 2017).

Types of Events

Considering the various types of events you might hold can help you select the one that best fits your current goals and resources. Charity walks, for example, are excellent for engaging large groups and promoting health and active living—and they come with the added benefit of being relatively easy to organize. Participants can raise funds through sponsorships or entry fees, and the event itself can serve as a platform for distributing educational materials about dementia. Gala dinners, on the other hand, are more formal and can be great for targeting higher-level donations. These events are opportune for speeches, auctions, and entertainment, all of which can come together to form an elegant atmosphere that encourages generous giving. These are just two of the dozens of options to choose from when planning your perfect community event.

Each event type offers unique benefits and challenges, so you should be aware of the pluses and hurdles you might encounter. For example, while charity walks can attract a high level of participation, they require careful route planning and coordination with local authorities for permits and security. Gala dinners, although potentially lucrative, involve significant upfront costs and detailed planning for catering, guest lists, and entertainment. Doing your research and considering the upsides and difficulties is how you can responsibly plan community events that make a true difference for those experiencing dementia.

Recruiting Volunteers

For community events, advocacy efforts, and fundraisers, it's likely that you'll benefit from recruiting volunteers, especially if the turnout is going to be more than a couple of people. Volunteers are able to provide the necessary manpower for everything from setting up the venue to managing the activities on the day of the event. You can work to recruit volunteers by communicating clearly about the event's purpose and the roles that volunteers are needed to fill. There are tons of places you can look for volunteers who are willing and passionate, including local community groups, schools, and online platforms.

Once volunteers are onboard, you also have to manage them as a part of leading a successful event. Clear instructions, proper training, and constant communication are all necessary if you want to be certain that volunteers are keeping everything in order. Assign roles to volunteers based on their strengths and interests to keep them motivated during the event. Don't forget to send out a thank-you after the event—doing so can help maintain their enthusiasm toward the cause and potentially secure their help with future events (Trish, n.d.).

Promotion and Marketing

Everything may be planned and ready to go, but there's one more thing to think about: promotion and marketing. Effective promotion and marketing are part of what guides your event to success, helping it reach its intended audience and achieve its goals. As we talked about with advocacy, you can promote and market your events by identifying the key messages you want to communicate and selecting the appropriate channels to reach your target audience. Local media outlets—like newspapers and bulletin boards—can be immensely valuable for promoting community events. You can also develop partnerships with local businesses and organizations to boost your promotional efforts. These connections can provide additional resources, extend your event's reach, and add credibility ("How to Promote a Fundraiser: Tips and Best Practices," n.d.).

THE IMPORTANCE OF PARTICIPATING IN RESEARCH

Advocacy and improving how people understand dementia doesn't have to extend solely to organizing events and campaigns. Participating in research related to early-onset dementia is a wonderful way to contribute to science and drive significant advancements in understanding and treatment. When you or a loved one chooses to become involved in research, you're helping to pave the way for breakthroughs that could benefit not only those currently affected by dementia but also future generations. Your help means adding to a growing body of knowledge that aims to refine diagnostic methods, develop more effective treatments, and ultimately improve the quality of life for those impacted by dementia.

The benefits of participating in research aren't solely scientific. For many, being part of a study brings a sense of purpose and contribution. Beyond that, research studies often offer participants access to the latest treatments before they are widely available, which can be particularly valuable when existing treatment options are limited. Moreover, participants in research studies are closely monitored, which can lead to a better understanding of their condition and individual health needs. This close observation can sometimes lead to insights about the disease that benefit the participant directly while still contributing to a broader understanding.

Finding Opportunities

If you're interested in participating in a research study, there are plenty of choices available both to people with dementia and their caregivers. Finding opportunities to participate in research can begin with contact points like local universities, hospitals, and research institutions known for their work in neurology and dementia. These spots often have ongoing studies and are usually looking for participants who can contribute to their research.

Another great choice for finding research opportunities is through online databases that list clinical trials and studies. Websites like ClinicalTrials.gov provide searchable listings of research studies around the world, which can be filtered by location, focus, and eligibility criteria. Engaging with patient advocacy groups and specialized dementia organizations can also provide leads on new research opportunities. These groups often have firsthand information on upcoming studies and can assist with the application and enrollment process.

Informed Consent

Understanding and obtaining informed consent is necessary when participating in any form of medical research. Having informed consent when participating in scientific research means that you have been informed of what the study does, what participation entails, the risks and benefits, and the rights you have as a participant—including the right to withdraw from the study at any time without penalty. It's essential that this information is communicated clearly and comprehensively so that you and your family can make well-informed decisions. Ethical standards that require studies to undergo rigorous ethical review and approval before they commence further guarantee that such studies adhere to internationally recognized scientific and ethical guidelines. Make sure to check that any study in which you want to participate meets these requirements (National Human Genome Research Institute 2022).

LEGISLATIVE ADVOCACY: HOW YOU CAN INFLUENCE DEMENTIA CARE POLICIES

As someone looking to advocate or become involved with improving the landscape for dementia patients on a wider scale, you might consider getting involved with legislative motions to influence care policies in a positive way. It can be daunting but rewarding simultaneously, and in order to do so, you should start with a firm understanding of how laws are made, amended, or repealed. Legislation related to dementia care typically progresses through several stages: introduction of a bill, committee review, debates, and then votes in both legislative chambers, followed by the executive's approval or veto. Advocates like you can significantly impact these motions at various stages, particularly during committee reviews where testimonies and expert opinions can sway the decisions of lawmakers. Engaging at the right moment with the right message can lead to meaningful changes in how dementia care is administered and funded, protecting the rights and improving the welfare of people with dementia as a result ("What Is Legislative Advocacy?," n.d.).

Lobbying

One way that you can play a hands-on role in shaping legislation, at least in the United States, is through lobbying, and believe it or not, effective lobbying is more than just persuading legislators. You can begin your journey with lobbying by identifying legislators who have shown interest in healthcare or, specifically, in aging and dementia-related issues. Reach out to these legislators with well-prepared briefs that include compelling data about the impact of dementia and the benefits of proposed changes or new policies. Personal stories from constituents can be particularly powerful in lobbying as well, as they put a human face on issues that might have previously been nothing more than data on a page to some legislators. When you meet with legislators or their staff, be clear, concise, and specific about what you are asking for and why it matters (Prosperity Now 2019).

Hearings and Consultations

Participating in public hearings and consultations is another effective way to influence dementia care policies. These forums create a platform for public input and are an opportunity to put dementia care issues on the legislative agenda. When preparing to speak at a hearing, be sure to focus on delivering a concise, impactful testimony that clearly outlines the problem, how it affects individuals and families, and what changes are needed to resolve this problem. Rehearse your statement to convey confidence and clarity and tweak it as needed, which will also make it easier for lawmakers to understand and support your position.

Keeping an Eye on Legislation

When you work to shape legislation, it is helpful to monitor and respond to changing legislation. Vigilance and a readiness to act are important making your voice heard in a timely way for prompt change. Stay informed about legislative developments that could affect dementia care by subscribing to updates from legislative tracking services or aligning with larger advocacy organizations that monitor these issues. Then, when action is needed, mobilize your community through social media campaigns, call-to-actions, or organizing letter-writing campaigns for legislators. Quick and coordinated responses—like being ready to speak up about the pitfalls of a change—can show strong public support for or opposition to proposed legislation, influencing lawmakers' decisions in the United States (Prosperity Now 2019).

As we move to the final leg of our journey together, remember that advocacy and community support come in all shapes and sizes. From raising awareness and educating the public to engaging with legislators and influencing policies, each action you take builds towards a more understanding and supportive society for those affected by early-onset dementia. The journey continues as we explore the next chapter, which delves into the essential resources and ongoing support available to navigate the challenges of dementia care. Together, these efforts weave a network of support that upholds the dignity and quality of life for individuals and families walking this path.

9

RESOURCES AND CONTINUING SUPPORT

No matter who you are and what your personal involvement is, being involved with dementia isn't sunshine and rainbows. Having the right resources, however, can make all the difference. This chapter is designed to help with precisely that—delivering a comprehensive repository of resources that will support, guide, and enlighten you through the various stages of dementia care right to your hands. Here, you'll find a carefully curated list of books, websites, hotlines, and organizations, each chosen for their relevance and helpfulness to your connection with dementia. Keep these resources on hand to help you when you need them.

COMPREHENSIVE DIRECTORY OF RESOURCES
FOR EARLY-ONSET DEMENTIA

Experiencing the journey of early-onset dementia requires access to a variety of resources that can provide support, information, and relief when you face challenges. To aid in this, take a look at this compilation of highly recommended resources:

- **Books:** For starters, books such as *The 36-Hour Day* by Nancy L. Mace and Peter V. Rabins offer invaluable advice on dealing with dementia.
- **Websites:** Websites like the Alzheimer's Association (alz.org) contain a wealth of information, including symptoms, stages, and care strategies, along with community forums where you can connect with others facing similar challenges.
- **Hotlines:** Hotlines are another excellent resource. They often include immediate assistance and support. For example, the Alzheimer's Association 24/7 Helpline (1-800-272-3900) allows you to speak with trained professionals who can provide advice, emotional support, and information on local resources.
- **Local Organizations:** For those seeking connection and community support, local organizations such as memory care clinics and regional Alzheimer's chapters are a great option. These organizations often offer support groups, educational workshops, and social events that can help reduce feelings of isolation and provide practical support.
- **Professionals:** Finding and connecting with medical and care specialists who have expertise in early-onset dementia is crucial. Your primary care physician can be a starting point for referrals to neurologists who specialize in dementia. Additionally, consider consulting with geriatric care managers who are trained to help navigate the complexities of dementia

care, from medical needs to coordinating in-home care services.
- **Government Organizations:** Government-based resources can also provide substantial support. Programs such as Medicaid may offer financial assistance for care services, for example.
- **Non-Profit Organizations:** Non-profit organizations can be helpful too. For instance, the National Institute on Aging (nia.nih.gov) has guides on symptoms, treatment options, and ongoing research. Non-profit organizations often provide services ranging from counseling to help with financial planning and legal advice.
- **International Support:** If you're reading this book from outside the U.S., it's important to explore dementia care resources available in your country. The Alzheimer's Disease International (ADI) website (alz.co.uk) is a good starting point, offering links to Alzheimer's associations worldwide. These associations can direct you to local resources, whether you are in the UK, Canada, Australia, or elsewhere.

Interactive Element: Resource Utilization Exercise

Create a list of your current challenges or questions related to dementia care. Next, using the options above or your own research, identify at least one resource that could help address each challenge or answer each question. This gives you a good starting point in understanding the resources available to you and how to use them.

CONTINUING EDUCATION: OPPORTUNITIES FOR LEARNING AND GROWTH

For some people, caregiving is something they research when they need a specific answer about a problem; however, caregiving and even being an advocate is improved when you stay informed and educated about dementia, even if certain concerns are no longer relevant to you. Staying informed about dementia and relevant social changes can empower you and strengthen your ability to provide compassionate and effective support for those with dementia.

Workshops and Seminars

You have tons of options when it comes to continuing your education on dementia. Educational workshops and seminars, for example, can be instrumental in the learning process. Events like these are usually hosted by healthcare professionals or dementia experts, and they focus on the latest techniques in dementia management and the newest research findings. For example, attending a workshop might provide you with insights into behavioral management strategies that are not widely known yet but have been proven effective in preliminary studies. These seminars also often have practical sessions where you can see dementia care techniques demonstrated firsthand, providing a clearer understanding than reading from a text.

Moreover, these workshops and seminars can be a platform for networking with other caregivers and professionals. This networking aspect can be incredibly beneficial—you can meet people who have faced similar challenges and can then work to exchange tips and solutions. These events are typically advertised through local hospitals, dementia care facilities, and community centers, and attending can be a refreshing reminder that you are not alone in this situation (Cherney 2021).

Online Courses and Webinars

Online courses and webinars present a flexible learning option that is particularly valuable if you have a tight schedule that makes attending in-person events challenging. For example, platforms like Coursera and Udemy have free or low-cost courses developed by medical professionals and universities, which you can attend from the comfort of your home. These courses range from understanding the basics of dementia to more advanced topics like neurocognitive disorders and their treatments. What's advantageous about online learning is the ability to pace your education according to your daily responsibilities. Additionally, many of these courses provide interactive forums where you can ask questions directly to experts or discuss topics with fellow learners, which can be enriching and informative, all while allowing for your daily rhythms to remain consistent ("Alzheimer's & Dementia Training & Education Center" 2019).

Community Classes

Local community classes are another excellent resource for continuous learning and engagement. Often offered by hospitals, universities, and community centers, these classes typically include topics such as nutritional planning for dementia patients, physical therapies to aid with mobility, or artistic activities that stimulate the mind. The local nature of these classes also means they are formulated around the specific resources and characteristics of your community, which can provide more relevant and immediately applicable knowledge. Furthermore, these classes mean that you can interact directly with those leading and other attendees, enforcing a community of local support that can be leaned on outside of class hours (Cherney 2021).

Self-Directed Learning

Finally, the importance of self-directed learning is significant and should be considered as you work with continuing your knowledge. In a field as ever-changing as dementia care, new discoveries and methodologies are continually surfacing. Engaging in self-directed learning by reading recent journals, books, and articles—or even watching YouTube videos for accessible learning—related to dementia care means that you can stay updated with the latest information. Participating actively in online forums dedicated to dementia care can also improve your understanding of dementia and help you access new coping mechanisms shared by others experiencing similar challenges.

INNOVATIONS IN DEMENTIA CARE: KEEPING UP-TO-DATE

How we treat, acknowledge, and manage dementia is always changing, especially in modern times, where technology and innovative care models are constantly being developed.

RESOURCES AND CONTINUING SUPPORT | 137

These innovations promise to enhance the quality of life for those living with the condition, and caregivers can benefit immensely from having an understanding of these advancements. When you stay up-to-date, not only can you support your loved one or yourself, but you can also contribute to supporting others.

Wearable technology, for instance, has positively shaped the way we monitor health in real time. Devices like smartwatches now come equipped with features that can track physiological information like heart rate and sleep patterns, and more importantly, they can detect irregularities that might indicate acute episodes or complications. This kind of technology means that we can adopt a more proactive and immediate method for health monitoring, where potential issues can be addressed before they escalate into serious problems.

Additionally, GPS tracking devices that can be embedded in clothing or accessories provide a layer of safety for people prone to wandering and peace of mind for their caregivers. These devices allow caregivers and families to monitor their loved ones' locations and receive alerts if they stray from safe zones. Previously, such advancements weren't available to us; taking advantage of those developments equates to better, more innovative care (Lifted Team 2019).

Innovations in Personalized Medicine

In the past, there was an attitude of treating each patient the same to provide equal care; now, however, the shift toward personalized medicine in dementia care is revolutionizing treatment paradigms through a lens of equity. Personalized medicine, as an approach, streamlines medical treatment to the individual characteristics of each patient based on their genetic profile, lifestyle, and environment. In the context of dementia, personalized medicine coincides with the potential to develop more effective management strategies that are specifically designed to suit the genetic makeup and unique needs of each person with the disease, potentially slowing the progression of the disease and improving overall outcomes as a result.

Integrated care pathways are another innovative model that enhances the coordination of services across different sectors and disciplines involved in dementia care. These pathways align various processes to be certain that all aspects of a patient's health are considered and addressed holistically, from medical treatment to social support and rehabilitation services. Integrated care pathways mean that no one area of your loved one's care is being neglected or undermined so that your loved one gets the care they need and deserve (Sullivan, Mannix, and Timmons 2017).

Research Breakthroughs

Another facet of remaining up-to-date, as mentioned earlier, is keeping an eye on research breakthroughs, especially if you're an advocate or someone with a loved one who has dementia. New research breakthroughs are being shaped daily, and they can notably improve our understanding and treatment of dementia in incredibly promising ways. These studies lead to new insights that could lead to better diagnostic tools and therapies as well. For example, studies exploring the role of tau proteins in neurodegeneration have opened new avenues for drug development, targeting specific pathways involved in the disease process (Alzheimer's Association 2021). Another exciting area of research is the use of artificial intelligence (AI) to identify patterns in brain imaging that precede the clinical symptoms of dementia, potentially leading to earlier and more accurate diagnoses ("Leveraging Artificial Intelligence for Healthy Aging and Dementia Research," n.d.).

Adapting to Innovations

Adapting to these innovations and integrating them into treatment options or healthcare plans requires you to remain flexible and informed. Integrating new technologies and care models into existing practices can be difficult, but the potential benefits for patient care are worth the effort. By staying informed about the latest developments in dementia care, attending workshops, and participating in training sessions that focus on new tools and methods, you have the power to elevate your caregiving techniques and improve the quality of life of those under your care.

In some cases, you might find that what works on paper might not work in the comfort of your own home. Research and theories are important, but evaluating their effectiveness and success in real-world settings is important. You should consider both the benefits and the drawbacks of each innovation you implement prior to doing so, including an assessment of whether a particular technology or treatment aligns with the needs and preferences of the person you are caring for. For example, while wearable technology options can provide valuable health data, it may not be right for all people with dementia who are wary of technology or prefer a higher degree of privacy.

BUILDING A SUSTAINABLE CAREGIVING NETWORK

Your knowledge and continued learning can be taken to the next level by building a sustainable caregiving network. Building a sustainable network for caregiving in the context of early-onset dementia involves seeking out support that encompasses family, friends, healthcare professionals, and community members. This network does far more than just share the load; it enriches the caregiving experience through emotional, practical, and professional support that can make a major difference in how you handle your daily responsibilities.

Initiating this network means reaching out actively—starting conversations, expressing needs clearly, and organizing regular meetings to ensure everyone involved is on the same page. Anyone you know—and some people who you don't—can be a part of this network. For example, engaging family members in open discussions about caregiving roles and expectations helps in distributing tasks in ways that fit each member's capacity and skills. Meanwhile, friends can offer respite and emotional support, stepping in to provide care or companionship that creates room for crucial breaks that rejuvenate your spirit and resilience. Moreover, integrating healthcare professionals into your network incorporates attention toward the medical and therapeutic needs of your loved one—which can then be met with exceptional precision and compassion.

Online Platforms

Just like online platforms can be used to help keep your loved one connected and to expand advocacy networks, online platforms have transformed how caregivers connect, learn, and support each other. Platforms like Alzheimer's Association forums and Facebook groups dedicated to dementia caregiving contain spaces where you can share experiences, exchange tips, and find emotional support from people who truly understand the challenges you face. This means that day or night, your questions can be answered, and your personal struggles as a caregiver can be met with compassion—something many caregivers overlook the need for in their quest to care for a loved one.

These digital communities are also instrumental in breaking the isolation often felt by caregivers. They mean that you can always find a shoulder to lean on or simply some advice about how to manage a new behavioral problem your loved one developed. Engaging with these online communities also allows you to stay updated on the latest caregiving strategies and medical advice, which can be directly applied to enhance your caregiving approach. The key to making the most of these platforms is active participation—asking questions, responding to others' queries, and sharing your own experiences candidly to keep the community alive.

Collaborative Caregiving

Collaborative caregiving is another aspect of building a sustainable network to consider. It involves working alongside others—such as other caregivers—to provide care to your loved one. One way to achieve this is by creating shared schedules with other caregivers to ensure your loved one receives continuous care while also balancing each caregiver's personal time and responsibilities. For instance, you might coordinate with a neighbor who also provides care to their loved one, trading hours or days when each of you can take breaks.

Additionally, engaging in co-caregiving strategies, where tasks are divided based on individual strengths and preferences, can make caregiving more manageable and effective. For example, one caregiver might be better at handling medical appointments while another excels at daily care routines. Recognizing and utilizing these strengths within your network enhances the quality of care and the overall well-being of both caregivers and the recipient of care.

Sustainable Caregiving

Sustainability in caregiving is important, too. It's more than immediate needs; sustainable caregiving also focuses on long-term practices that confirm that the network remains robust and responsive. Regular meetings with your caregiving network, whether in person or virtually, help review the care strategy, discuss any challenges, and readjust roles as needed, all of which set sustainability in stone. Clear, open communication is the lifeblood of these meetings, creating an environment where everyone involved has a voice and any issues are addressed promptly and effectively. Establishing mutual support agreements, where caregivers commit to supporting each other's health and well-being, can also strengthen your network. These agreements might include commitments to step in when another caregiver feels overwhelmed or to share resources like information about new treatment practices or caregiving tools ("What Are Some Effective Strategies to Build and Maintain a Strong Caregiver Network?" n.d.).

THE FUTURE OF DEMENTIA CARE: TRENDS AND PREDICTIONS

As we look to the future of dementia care, we are already noticing that an interesting shift is underway—one of empathy, dignity, and support for people with dementia. A notable trend in the landscape of care, for example, is the increasing move towards home-based care (Luísa Pelucio et al. 2023). This trend is the result of our understanding of the therapeutic benefits of familiar environments on the mental and emotional well-being of people with dementia. Home-based care, beyond familiarity, allows for personalized attention and a unique care routine, both of which are crucial in managing the day-to-day challenges of dementia. Furthermore, it enables continuous family involvement, which is not only comforting for the person with dementia but also provides family members with greater oversight and participation in the care process.

In tandem with the shift towards home-based settings, there's a rising emphasis on holistic care approaches. Such approaches integrate physical, psychological, and social aspects of care to provide comprehensive support that addresses the multifaceted needs of dementia patients. Holistic care might include activities like music therapy, which has been shown to help manage stress and evoke memories, or pet therapy, which can increase social interaction and physical activity. These therapies are becoming more integrated into care plans as we develop a broader understanding of health that includes emotional and social well-being, not just physical health ("Everything You Need to Know about Holistic Dementia Care! - Family Medicine & Geriatric Center" 2023).

There are new breakthroughs in medical research that could significantly alter the course of dementia treatment. Researchers are exploring the potential of gene therapy as a way to directly address the genetic factors that contribute to dementia. These studies may very well indicate that hope is on the horizon, not just treatment but potentially the prevention of dementia altogether (Levy, 2023). Similarly, advances in biomarker technology also hold promise when it comes to the potential to enhance diagnostic accuracy and allow for earlier intervention, which can be vital in managing the disease's progression ("Biomarker Research," n.d.).

Understanding the trends and predictions surrounding dementia treatment and care equips you with the knowledge that can improve how you interact with those you care for. Simultaneously, these changes lead to a sense of hope and action both for you as a caregiver and for people who receive early-onset dementia diagnoses in the future. Being open to new methods and ideas that could significantly enhance the quality of care and life for those experiencing early-onset dementia is equally as important as the developments themselves. As we continue to witness and contribute to these advancements, the landscape of dementia care is reshaped, bringing new solutions and greater hope to families navigating this challenging condition. You can integrate these solutions into your approach, and as you do, remember that each step forward can make a massive difference in the lives of people with dementia and their families.

REVIEWING AND REVISING CARE PLANS: AN ONGOING PROCESS

We've talked about it a few times before, but I can't really overstate just how important it is for care plans to be reviewed and revised regularly. As you well know, the progression of early-onset dementia is not linear—people progress at different rates, and each set of skills, from cognitive to physical, can progress at different rates, too. These changes can be rapid or slow-acting, and adjustments in your care strategies are often necessary to meet the shifting needs of your loved one.

Regularly revisiting the care plan means that you can assert that every aspect of care is still effective and appropriate, and if it's not, it can be adapted to meet changes in health status, integrate advancements in medical treatments, or respect your loved one's new preferences and behaviors. This process of reviewing and revising your loved one's care plan is a necessary component of providing responsive and compassionate care that truly meets the needs of your loved one with dementia.

Reviewing the Care Plan

When working on a review of your loved one's care plan, you should have their entire care team present, including you, their primary caregiver (if that isn't you), other family members, doctors, nurses, and possibly in-home care professionals if they're involved. Each member of this team brings a unique perspective to the table and can communicate valuable information based on their personal interactions and experiences with the person with dementia. For instance, a family member might notice subtle changes in behavior that could indicate a need for adjustment in mental health strategies, while a healthcare professional might suggest modifications based on the latest treatment advancements.

Your loved one should be as involved in this process as possible because, after all, it's *their* care being discussed. Also, despite the challenges of dementia, they may still be able to express their preferences and discomforts, which should guide the adjustments in the care plan for as long as possible. If they can't communicate these things, legal documentation like a living will or DPOA should be considered when making care plan changes.

Adjusting Based on the Review

The process of adjusting care strategies based on the findings of your review has to be managed with precision. If your loved one's cognitive abilities have declined, for example, they might benefit from increased supervision or more structured daily routines to ensure their safety and well-being, and the revised care plan should reflect this. Alternatively, if a new study suggests that a different approach or therapy could be more effective for your loved one's particular case, integrating this into the care plan might provide better outcomes. Potential adjustments might also include introducing new activities that align with your loved one's current interests and abilities.

Documentation and Record Keeping

Throughout this process, keeping records and documenting changes and progress is important to continue to make informed, cohesive decisions based on the effectiveness of various care strategies, and any challenges encountered are invaluable. These records inform future review progress while assisting you when it comes to tracking how your loved one's dementia is progressing. Playing a role in helping maintain thorough and up-to-date records shapes each member of the care team's understanding as well, leading to better decisions and the ability of everyone to be on the same page.

NURTURING HOPE AND POSITIVITY IN THE FACE OF DEMENTIA

As you strive to work through everything involved in managing early-onset dementia, maintaining a positive outlook might sometimes feel just as difficult as managing the physical symptoms of the condition itself. It's in these moments that a mindset focused on hope and positivity can be most beneficial. Caregiving can wear you down if you aren't taking the time to infuse your practices with positivity. For example, take advantage of a perspective that focuses on celebrating small victories each day, as it can significantly influence your emotional and mental well-being. These victories might be as simple as sharing a smile during a morning walk or enjoying a moment of clarity in conversation. Such instances, though small, are immense triumphs that highlight the high spirits of your loved one and your dedication to their care.

Additionally, fusing humor into daily interactions can be a great way to lighten the mood and atmosphere, making space for joy and laughter that uplifts both you and your loved one each and every day. Humor can also be a window back to the person your loved one was before dementia began to take hold, reminding you both of happier times and strengthening your connection in the process.

It's also a great idea to read, listen to, or seek out inspirational stories of caregivers and those with dementia to keep you and your loved one feeling hopeful and motivated. Hearing or reading about individuals and families who have walked similar paths can be incredibly uplifting. For example, I once knew a man who, despite his diagnosis, took up painting—a hobby he had never before attempted. His artwork was filled with vibrant colors and bold artistic choices, and it quickly became his favorite way to express himself when words failed him. This brought great joy to his family and friends and inspired me to integrate creativity into the care of my own loved one. Stories like these highlight the resilience and creativity that can flourish in those with dementia, even in the face of dementia's challenges. There are always opportunities for growth and joy, and inspirational stories remind us of this.

If you or your family is spiritual or religious, then you can further boost your positivity and healthy mindset by integrating those beliefs into your daily routines. Spirituality or faith often does a lot in the way of providing comfort and resilience, both for those experiencing dementia and for their caregivers. For many people, spiritual beliefs and practices lead to a strong sense of peace and purpose, which can be anchoring during times of uncertainty. Whether it's prayer, meditation, or attending religious services, these spiritual- and faith-based habits can grant you a reprieve from the daily stresses and emotional turmoil of dementia caregiving. They can also be a source of community support since many religious and spiritual practices come along with the added benefit of a community that shares similar values and experiences and who can offer empathy and understanding. Engaging in spiritual activities together with your loved one can also be a comforting ritual that strengthens your relationship and sense of togetherness with one another.

Finally, be sure to take advantage of resources like the ones provided to you earlier when it comes to prompting hope and positivity in your life and that of your loved one. It can be easy to feel like you're braving the path of dementia all on your own, but websites, organizations, support groups, and even governmental assistance can fill gaps where you feel down or unsure of where to go. From emotional support to the financial and practical assistance needed to help you maintain confidence, taking advantage of the abundant dementia-related resources can be your saving grace during such a tricky time.

REFLECTIONS AND NEXT STEPS FOR CAREGIVERS AND PATIENTS

Before we close out our journey together, I want to highlight the importance of taking a moment to pause and reflect on your experiences as a caregiver or a patient dealing with early-onset dementia—it's something that can be incredibly grounding and insightful. It allows you to appreciate the strides you've made, recognize the hurdles you've overcome, and consider adjustments that might enhance your journey forward. As you reflect, think about the strategies, routines, and interactions that have worked well. What brought moments of joy and connection? What seemed to ease the challenges on particularly tough days? Such reflection can reinforce effective practices and boost your confidence in handling future challenges.

Conversely, consider what might need adjustment either in your own life or the life of your loved one. Are there aspects of care that have become more challenging or less effective? Perhaps certain activities that once brought enjoyment no longer have an impact in the same way, or maybe communication strategies need to be tweaked as needs evolve—such as simplifying methods or helping your loved one communicate non-verbally.

It's also beneficial to set realistic goals for the future. For caregivers, this might look like finding more time for self-care or learning new caregiving skills. For people with dementia, goals can focus on maintaining certain physical activities or social interactions that boost well-being. Setting these goals together, where possible, can bring meaning and the chance for achievement alongside a sense of mutual support and connection.

It's also important to consider what the road ahead might look like if you're a caregiver. I don't mean the immediate next steps, but rather how you'll adjust and cope after caregiving is no longer a necessary part of your life. It can be a huge emotional shift and leave you feeling at a loss when such a constant responsibility is no longer present in your life. Seeking therapy or grief counseling services can help get your mental health back on track, as can finding activities to fill your day. You can even make strides to help others—either with dementia or their caregivers—to pass along the wisdom and fulfillment you've gained during your time as a caregiver.

Embracing the role of mentorship can be a fulfilling next step for experienced caregivers. If you've managed the complexities of dementia care for some time, or if you're looking for a way to fill a gap after caregiving duties are no longer needed, consider mentoring someone who is new to this journey. Sharing your insights, strategies, and encouragement can dramatically ease the stress for novice caregivers. It also creates a supportive community that improves the collective resilience and knowledge surrounding caregiving. Mentorship does not require formal arrangements; it can be as simple as offering to be a listening ear, sharing resources, or providing practical tips based on your experiences.

CONCLUSION

As we draw close to the end of our journey together through the pages of this book, I want to take a moment to reflect on the ground we have covered and the shared path we have walked in understanding and managing early-onset dementia. From understanding the fundamentals of this condition and traversing the complexities of legal and financial planning to making daily adjustments and embracing emotional support, our exploration has been deep and wide-ranging. We've reviewed practical caregiving strategies and highlighted the immense power of quality-of-life enhancements through therapeutic activities, community involvement, and meticulous advanced care planning, and each consideration has led you to a better place of understanding whether you have dementia yourself or seek to care for a loved one.

Dementia can often be an isolating, challenging experience, but if you only glean one thing from this book, let it be this: Despite the undeniable challenges posed by early-onset dementia, there are abundant opportunities to enrich the lives of those affected. By taking the time to engage in meaningful activities, fostering community connections, and planning thoughtfully for the future, people like you and I can illuminate the path of dementia treatment and caregiving not just with hope but with joy and fulfillment, too.

I urge you to continue educating yourself and stay on top of the latest developments in dementia care. As we've discussed, the terrain of this field is ever-evolving, and remaining adaptable allows you to integrate new knowledge and resources into your care strategies effectively. And remember, the strength of a support network can't be overlooked if you hope to offer quality of life and meaningful care to those with dementia. Building and sustaining a network of family, friends, healthcare professionals, and online communities is essential.

Let this book serve as your sign to take proactive, hands-on steps in your dementia care journey. Whether it's applying the strategies we've discussed, joining or forming support groups, participating in research, or advocating for policy changes, your active participation makes a big difference in improving the quality of life for your loved one and improving the medical and social supports for people who will develop dementia in the future. Every small step you take is a leap forward in terms of supporting those with this disease.

Before we part ways, I wanted to thank you from the bottom of my heart for committing yourself to caring for someone with early-onset dementia. Not everyone is willing to step up to the plate, but your commitment is truly awe-inspiring. Your journey is marked by challenges, but more importantly, it is defined by your strength, compassion, and unwavering dedication. You are not alone in this; our solidarity is a light that shines brighter with each shared experience and learned insight, so never be afraid to lean on others for support on your path.

Through our collective efforts, we are paving the way toward significant advancements in dementia care. Each challenge we encounter is not a setback but a way to forge deeper connections, to learn, and to grow. Together, we are not just facing early-onset dementia; we are actively shaping a world where every person affected by this condition can live with dignity, respect, and joy. Thank you for being a part of this meaningful journey.

BIBLIOGRAPHY

"5 Benefits of Swimming for Seniors Who Need Alzheimer's Care | Richmond West." n.d. Www.seniorhelpers.com. https://www.seniorhelpers.com/va/greater-richmond/resources/blogs/5-benefits-of-swimming-for-seniors-who-need-alzheimers-care-richmond/#:~

"6 Dehydration Facts That May Surprise You." n.d. Drip Drop ORS. https://www.dripdrop.com/blog/health-wellness/6-dehydration-facts-may-surprise.

"6 Ways That Art Therapy Can Help People with Memory Loss | Lesley University." n.d. Lesley.edu. https://lesley.edu/article/6-ways-that-art-therapy-can-help-people-with-memory-loss.

"7 Dementia Friendly Kitchen Appliances & Devices." 2022. DementiaWho! May 19, 2022. https://dementiawho.com/dementia-friendly-kitchen-appliances/.

"8 Ways Walking Can Boost Your Brain Health." n.d. ER of Texas. https://www.eroftexas.com/8-ways-walking-can-boost-your-brain-health/#:~

"A Sharper Mind: Tai Chi Can Improve Cognitive Function." 2020. Harvard Health. January 16, 2020. https://www.health.harvard.edu/mind-and-mood/a-sharper-mind-tai-chi-can-improve-cognitive-function#:~:

"Alzheimer's & Dementia Training & Education Center." 2019. Alz.org. 2019. https://training.alz.org/.

Alzheimer's Association. 2020. "Daily Care Plan." Alzheimer's Disease and Dementia. 2020. https://www.alz.org/help-support/caregiving/daily-care/daily-care-plan.

———. 2021. "Tau." https://www.alz.org/media/documents/alzheimers-dementia-tau-ts.pdf.

———. 2022. "10 Early Signs and Symptoms of Alzheimer's." Alzheimer's Disease and Dementia. Alzheimer's Association. 2022. https://www.alz.org/alzheimers-dementia/10_signs.

———. 2023. "Medical Tests." Alzheimer's Disease and Dementia. 2023. https://www.alz.org/alzheimers-dementia/diagnosis/medical_tests#:~

Alzheimer's Society. 2019. "Recognising When Someone Is Reaching the End of Their Life." Alzheimer's Society. 2019. https://www.alzheimers.

org.uk/get-support/help-dementia-care/recognising-when-someone-reaching-end-their-life.

——. 2022. "The Psychological and Emotional Impact of Dementia." Alzheimer's Society. June 27, 2022. https://www.alzheimers.org.uk/get-support/help-dementia-care/understanding-supporting-person-dementia-psychological-emotional-impact.

Anderson, Merryn, Rachel Menon, Katy Oak, and Louise Allan. 2022. "The Use of Technology for Social Interaction by People with Dementia: A Scoping Review." Edited by Matthew Chua Chin Heng. *PLOS Digital Health* 1 (6): e0000053. https://doi.org/10.1371/journal.pdig.0000053.

Awada, Adnan A. 2015. "Early and Late-Onset Alzheimer's Disease: What Are the Differences?" *Journal of Neurosciences in Rural Practice* 6 (03): 455–56. https://doi.org/10.4103/0976-3147.154581.

Baig, Edward C. 2023. "5 Ways Tech Can Help Caregivers of Dementia Patients." AARP. AARP. May 2023. https://www.aarp.org/home-family/personal-technology/info-2023/dementia-caregiver-technology.html.

Banerjee, S. 2006. "Quality of Life in Dementia: More than Just Cognition. An Analysis of Associations with Quality of Life in Dementia." *Journal of Neurology, Neurosurgery & Psychiatry* 77 (2): 146–48. https://doi.org/10.1136/jnnp.2005.072983.

BAYADA Home Health Care. 2019. "What Is Spiritual Care in Hospice?" Be Healthy Blog. 2019. https://blog.bayada.com/be-healthy/what-is-spiritual-care-in-hospice#:~:.

Better Health Channel. 2014. "Dementia - Early Signs." Vic.gov.au. May 31, 2014. https://www.betterhealth.vic.gov.au/health/conditionsandtreatments/dementia-early-signs.

——. 2021. "Exercise and Mental Health." Better Health Channel. December 20, 2021. https://www.betterhealth.vic.gov.au/health/healthyliving/exercise-and-mental-health.

"Biomarker Research." n.d. National Institute on Aging. https://www.nia.nih.gov/report-2020-2021-scientific-advances-prevention-treatment-and-care-dementia/biomarker-research.

"Caring for a Person with Late-Stage Alzheimer's Disease." 2021. National Institute on Aging. May 27, 2021. https://www.nia.nih.gov/health/alzheimers-caregiving/caring-person-late-stage-alzheimers-disease.

Cherney, Kristeen. 2021. "Alzheimer's Support Group: Near You, Online, and More." Healthline. August 5, 2021. https://www.healthline.com/health/alzheimers/alzheimers-support-group.

Desai, Nirali. 2024. "Useful Dementia Apps for Seniors and Their Care-

BIBLIOGRAPHY | 159

givers." Www.aplaceformom.com. 2024. https://www.aplaceformom.com/caregiver-resources/articles/dementia-apps.

"Diet and Dementia | Alzheimer's Society." n.d. Www.alzheimers.org.uk. Accessed June 28, 2024. https://www.alzheimers.org.uk/about-dementia/managing-the-risk-of-dementia/additional-treatments-for-dementia-risk/diet#:~

Dighriri, Ibrahim M., Abdalaziz M. Alsubaie, Fatimah M. Hakami, Dalal M. Hamithi, Maryam M. Alshekh, Fatimah A. Khobrani, Fatimah E. Dalak, et al. 2022. "Effects of Omega-3 Polyunsaturated Fatty Acids on Brain Functions: A Systematic Review." *Cureus* 14 (10). https://doi.org/10.7759/cureus.30091.

"Does Long-Term Care Insurance Cover Memory Care? A Comprehensive Guide." 2023. The National Council on Aging. 2023. https://www.ncoa.org/article/does-long-term-care-insurance-cover-memory-care-a-comprehensive-guide.

Durán-Gómez, Noelia, Jorge Guerrero-Martín, Demetrio Pérez-Civantos, Casimiro Fermín López Jurado, Patricia Palomo-López, and Macarena C Cáceres. 2020. "Understanding Resilience Factors among Caregivers of People with Alzheimer's Disease in Spain." *Psychology Research and Behavior Management* Volume 13 (November): 1011–25. https://doi.org/10.2147/prbm.s274758.

Dyk, Deirdre van, and Linda Dono. 2017. "Caregivers Creating a Safe Home for Those with Dementia." AARP. December 2017. https://www.aarp.org/caregiving/home-care/info-2017/dementia-home-safety.html.

"Educational Programs and Dementia Care Resources." 2021. Alzheimer's Disease and Dementia. 2021. https://www.alz.org/help-support/resources/care-education-resources.

"Eligibility Guidelines | Passages Hospice | Louisiana." n.d. Passages Hospice. Accessed June 30, 2024. https://passages-hospice.com/eligibility/#:~

"Everything You Need to Know about Holistic Dementia Care! - Family Medicine & Geriatric Center." 2023. Family Medicine & Geriatric Center. January 4, 2023. https://fmgcenter.com/everything-you-need-to-know-about-holistic-dementia-care/#:~

"Exercise Can Boost Your Memory and Thinking Skills." 2023. Harvard Health. October 20, 2023. https://www.health.harvard.edu/mind-and-mood/exercise-can-boost-your-memory-and-thinking-skills#:~

Family Caregiver Alliance. 2016. "Caregiver's Guide to Understanding Dementia Behaviors." Family Caregiver Alliance. 2016. https://www.caregiver.org/resource/caregivers-guide-understanding-dementia-behaviors/.

Fayaz, Imran. 2016. "How Dehydration Affects Your Brain - the Brain & Spine Institute of North Houston." Imran Fayaz. February 16, 2016. https://fayazneurosurgery.com/how-dehydration-affects-your-brain/#:~

"Finalizing Your Durable Power of Attorney for Finances." n.d. Www.willmaker.com. Accessed July 9, 2024. https://www.willmaker.com/legal-manual/durable-powers-of-attorney-for-finances/finalizing-your-durable-power-of-attorney-for-finances.html#:~

"Financial and Legal Planning for Caregivers." 2023. Alzheimer's Disease and Dementia. 2023. https://www.alz.org/help-support/caregiving/financial-legal-planning.

"Frequently Asked Questions about Durable Powers of Attorney for Health Care." n.d. Www.lawhelp.org. https://www.lawhelp.org/dc/resource/frequently-asked-questions-about-durable-powe#:~

Friedman, Esther M, Thomas E Trail, Christine Anne Vaughan, and Terri Tanielian. 2018. "Online Peer Support Groups for Family Caregivers: Are They Reaching the Caregivers with the Greatest Needs?" *Journal of the American Medical Informatics Association* 25 (9): 1130–36. https://doi.org/10.1093/jamia/ocy086.

"Getting Treatment for Depression, Anxiety or Apathy." n.d. Www.alzheimers.org.uk. https://www.alzheimers.org.uk/about-dementia/symptoms-and-diagnosis/talking-therapies#:~

Gordon, Sherri. 2024. "6 Characteristics Every Power of Attorney Should Have." Verywell Health. 2024. https://www.verywellhealth.com/characteristics-for-choosing-power-of-attorney-4134991#:~

"Hobbies and Dementia Craftivism." n.d. Https://Livingwithdementiatoolkit.org.uk/. https://livingwithdementiatoolkit.org.uk/keep-a-sense-of-purpose/hobbies-and-dementia-craftivism/#:~

"Home Safety." 2021. Alzheimer's Disease and Dementia. 2021. https://www.alz.org/help-support/caregiving/safety/home-safety#:~

"How Can I Find Memory Care near Me?" 2018. A Place for Mom. 2018. https://www.aplaceformom.com/alzheimers-care.

"How to Promote a Fundraiser: Tips and Best Practices." n.d. Mailchimp. https://mailchimp.com/resources/how-to-promote-a-fundraiser/.

"How to Provide Additional Comfort at End of Life." 2022. Www.crossroadshospice.com. 2022. https://www.crossroadshospice.com/hospice-palliative-care-blog/2022/may/25/how-to-provide-additional-comfort-at-end-of-life/.

Hung, Lillian, Allison Hudson, Mario Gregorio, Lynn Jackson, Jim Mann, Neil Horne, Annette Berndt, Christine Wallsworth, Lily Wong, and Alison Phinney. 2021. "Creating Dementia-Friendly Communities for Social Inclusion: A Scoping Review." *Gerontology and Geriatric Medicine* 7 (January): 233372142110135. https://doi.org/10.1177/23337214211013596.

"Inside the Brain." 2020. Alzheimer's Disease and Dementia. 2020. https://www.alz.org/alzheimers-dementia/what-is-alzheimers/brain_tour_part_2#:~

"Is It Dementia or Depression?" 2021. Harvard Health. May 1, 2021. https://www.health.harvard.edu/mind-and-mood/is-it-dementia-or-depression#:~

Keene, Valerie. 2022. "How to Write a Living Will." Www.nolo.com. 2022. https://www.nolo.com/legal-encyclopedia/how-write-living-will.html.

Lennon, Emma. n.d. "Best Home Automation Ideas and Technology to Help with Dementia Care." Homage Australia. Accessed July 9, 2024. https://www.homage.com.au/resources/dementia-home-automation/#:~:

"Leveraging Artificial Intelligence for Healthy Aging and Dementia Research." n.d. National Institute on Aging. Accessed June 30, 2024. https://www.nia.nih.gov/artificial-intelligence#:~

Levy, Brandon. 2023. "Gene Therapy Protects Neurons from Alzheimer's Disease | NIH Intramural Research Program." Irp.nih.gov. 2023. https://irp.nih.gov/blog/post/2023/12/gene-therapy-protects-neurons-from-alzheimers-disease.

Lifted Team. 2019. "Tracking Devices and Dementia: What You Need to Know." Lifted. November 28, 2019. https://www.liftedcare.com/news/tracking-devices-and-dementia-what-you-need-to-know/#:~

Long, Annabelle, Claudio Di Lorito, Pip Logan, Vicky Booth, Louise Howe, Vicky Hood-Moore, and Veronika van der Wardt. 2020. "The Impact of a Dementia-Friendly Exercise Class on People Living with Dementia: A Mixed-Methods Study." *International Journal of Environmental Research and Public Health* 17 (12): 4562. https://doi.org/10.3390/ijerph17124562.

Luísa Pelucio, Cristina Nascimento, Laiana A Quagliato, and Antônio Egídio Nardi. 2023. "Home Care for the Elderly with Dementia: A Systematic Review." *Dementia & Neuropsychologia* 17 (January). https://doi.org/10.1590/1980-5764-dn-2022-0052.

"Managing Personality and Behavior Changes in Alzheimer's." 2017. National Institute on Aging. May 17, 2017. https://www.nia.nih.gov/

health/alzheimers-changes-behavior-and-communication/managing-personality-and-behavior-changes.

Mayo Clinic. 2023. "Dementia - Symptoms and Causes." Mayo Clinic. August 30, 2023. https://www.mayoclinic.org/diseases-conditions/dementia/symptoms-causes/syc-20352013.

"Medicare Enrollment Numbers." 2023. Center for Medicare Advocacy. January 12, 2023. https://medicareadvocacy.org/medicare-enrollment-numbers/.

Mendez, Mario F. 2019. "Early-Onset Alzheimer Disease and Its Variants." CONTINUUM: Lifelong Learning in Neurology 25 (1): 34–51. https://doi.org/10.1212/con.0000000000000687.

"MIND and Mediterranean Diets Linked to Fewer Signs of Alzheimer's Brain Pathology." 2023. National Institute on Aging. May 4, 2023. https://www.nia.nih.gov/news/mind-and-mediterranean-diets-linked-fewer-signs-alzheimers-brain-pathology.

Momand, Beheshta, Olivia Sacuevo, Masuoda Hamidi, Winnie Sun, and Adam Dubrowski. 2022. "Using Communication Accommodation Theory to Improve Communication between Healthcare Providers and Persons with Dementia." Cureus 14 (10). https://doi.org/10.7759/cureus.30618.

National Human Genome Research Institute. 2022. "Why Is Informed Consent Required?" Genome.gov. January 3, 2022. https://www.genome.gov/about-genomics/educational-resources/fact-sheets/why-is-informed-consent-required.

NHS. 2023. "How to Get a Dementia Diagnosis." Nhs.uk. August 18, 2023. https://www.nhs.uk/conditions/dementia/symptoms-and-diagnosis/diagnosis/#:~

OneCause. 2017. "Planning a Successful Fundraising Event in 10 Steps: The Updated Guide." OneCause. March 1, 2017. https://www.onecause.com/blog/fundraising-event-planning/.

"Palliative Care and Dementia." n.d. Get Palliative Care. https://getpalliativecare.org/whatis/disease-types/dementia-palliative-care/.

"Participating in Alzheimer's Disease and Related Dementias Research." n.d. National Institute on Aging. https://www.nia.nih.gov/health/clinical-trials-and-studies/participating-alzheimers-disease-and-related-dementias-research.

"Preparing a Living Will." 2022. National Institute on Aging. October 31, 2022. https://www.nia.nih.gov/health/advance-care-planning/preparing-living-will.

Prosperity Now. 2019. "How Do I Advocate for Policy Change? | Prosperity Now." Prosperitynow.org. 2019. https://prosperitynow.org/putting-prosperity-within-reach-how-do-i-advocate-for-policy-change.

"Setting Routines and Reminders." n.d. Alzheimer Society of Canada. https://alzheimer.ca/en/help-support/im-caring-person-living-dementia/providing-day-day-care/setting-routines-reminders.

Stanborough, Rebecca. 2020. "How to Find a Therapist That's Right for You: 9 Key Tips." Healthline. August 17, 2020. https://www.healthline.com/health/how-to-find-a-therapist.

"Stigma against Dementia." n.d. Alzheimer Society of Canada. https://alzheimer.ca/en/about-dementia/stigma-against-dementia.

Sullivan, Dawn O., Mary Mannix, and Suzanne Timmons. 2017. "Integrated Care Pathways and Care Bundles for Dementia in Acute Care: Concept versus Evidence." *American Journal of Alzheimer's Disease & Other Dementiasr* 32 (4): 189–93. https://doi.org/10.1177/1533317517698791.

"The Role of Personalized Healthcare." 2024. ChartSpan. April 23, 2024. https://www.chartspan.com/blog/the-role-of-personalized-healthcare/#:~

"The Unexpected Benefits of Music Therapy for Dementia Patient." 2023. Pacific Neuroscience Institute. September 12, 2023. https://www.pacificneuroscienceinstitute.org/blog/dementia/the-unexpected-benefits-of-music-therapy-for-dementia-patients-according-to-a-geriatrician/.

Trish. n.d. "7 Ways to Boost Volunteer Recruitment in Your Nonprofit." Springly. https://www.springly.org/en-us/blog/volunteer-recruitment-nonprofit/.

Tyrrell, Patrick, Seneca Harberger, Caroline Schoo, and Waquar Siddiqui. 2023. "Kubler-Ross Stages of Dying and Subsequent Models of Grief." National Library of Medicine. StatPearls Publishing. February 26, 2023. https://www.ncbi.nlm.nih.gov/books/NBK507885/.

U.S. Department Of Labor. 2024. "Americans with Disabilities Act | U.S. Department of Labor." Www.dol.gov. 2024. https://www.dol.gov/general/topic/disability/ada#:~

"Understanding the Differences between Palliative and Hospice Care." n.d. Alzheimer's Foundation of America. Accessed June 30, 2024. https://alzfdn.org/understanding-differences-palliative-hospice-care/.

"Virtually Support World Alzheimer's Month." n.d. Alzheimer's Disease International. https://www.alzint.org/news-events/news/virtually-support-world-alzheimers-month/#:~

"What Are Some Effective Strategies to Build and Maintain a Strong Caregiver Network?" n.d. Www.linkedin.com. Accessed July 9, 2024. https://www.linkedin.com/advice/0/what-some-effective-strategies-build-maintain-strong.

"What Are the Signs of Alzheimer's Disease?" n.d. National Institute on Aging. https://www.nia.nih.gov/health/alzheimers-symptoms-and-diagnosis/what-are-signs-alzheimers-disease#:~

"What Do We Know about Diet and Prevention of Alzheimer's Disease?" n.d. National Institute on Aging. https://www.nia.nih.gov/health/alzheimers-and-dementia/what-do-we-know-about-diet-and-prevention-alzheimers-disease#:~:

"What Is Dementia?" 2022. Alzheimer's Disease and Dementia. 2022. https://www.alz.org/alzheimers-dementia/what-is-dementia#:~:

"What Is Dementia? Symptoms, Types, and Diagnosis." 2022. National Institute on Aging. December 8, 2022. https://www.nia.nih.gov/health/alzheimers-and-dementia/what-dementia-symptoms-types-and-diagnosis#:~:

"What Is Legislative Advocacy?" n.d. https://tcadp.org/wp-content/uploads/2010/07/Legislative-Advocacy-101.pdf.

"What Is Memory Care?" 2023. NCOA Adviser. 2023. https://www.ncoa.org/adviser/local-care/memory-care/#:~

"What to Look for When Searching for a Memory Care Facility." 2021. StoneBridge Senior Living. November 3, 2021. https://stonebridgeseniorliving.com/what-to-look-for-when-searching-for-a-memory-care-facility/#:~

"What's Medicare Supplement Insurance (Medigap)? | Medicare." n.d. Www.medicare.gov. https://www.medicare.gov/health-drug-plans/medigap.

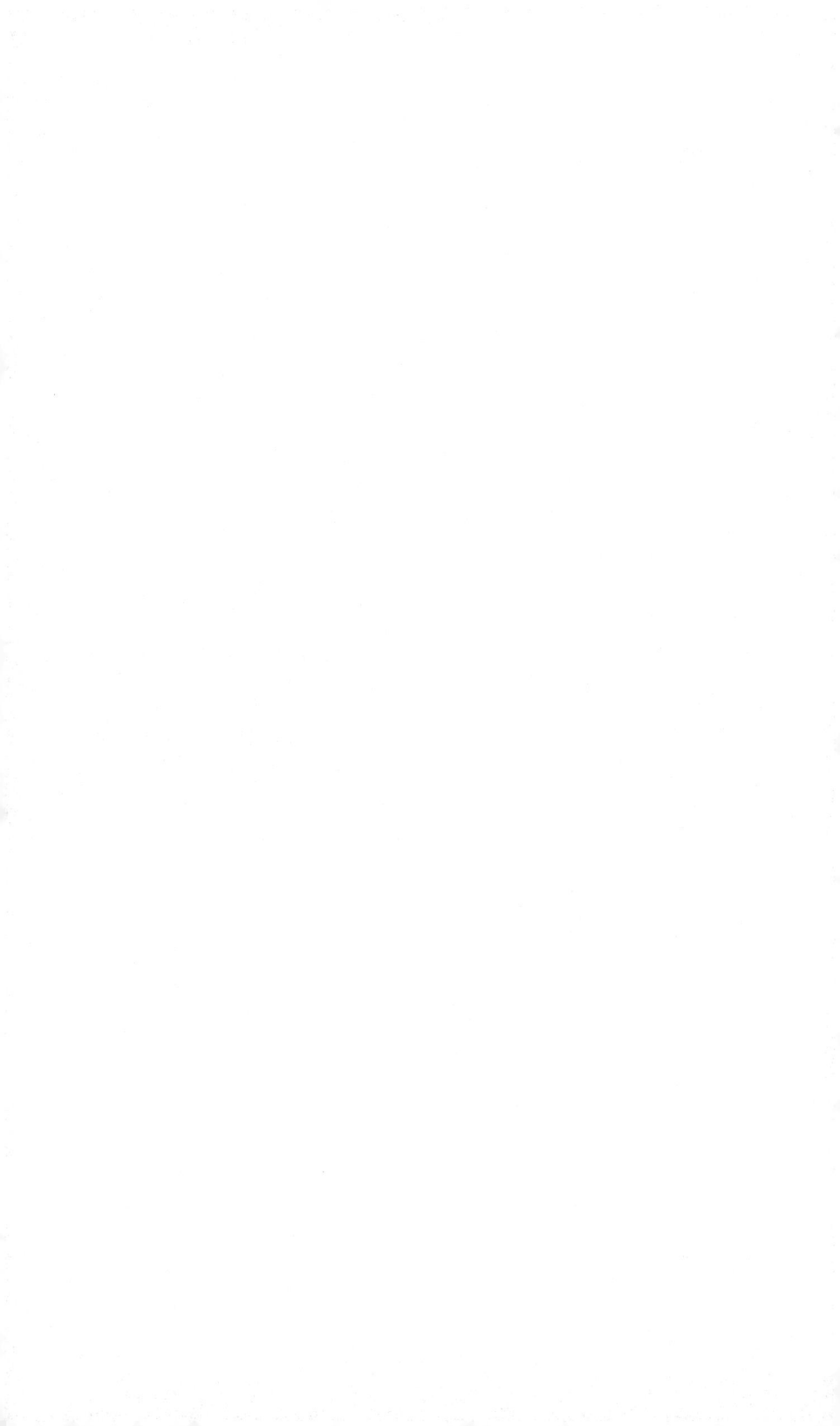

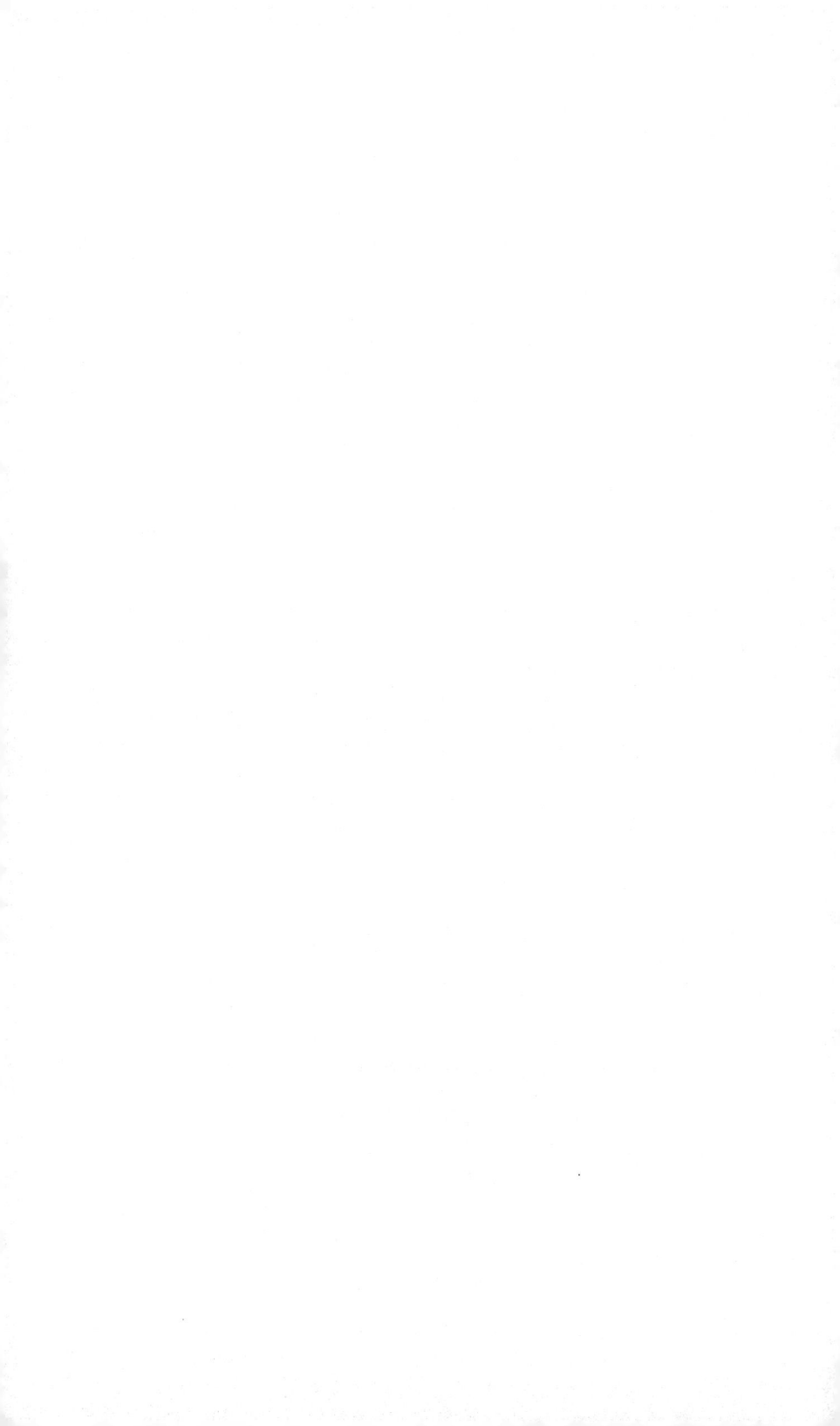

Made in the USA
Las Vegas, NV
15 September 2024